Intrapartum Care for the MRCOG and Beyond

Second edition

Published titles in the MRCOG and Beyond series

Antenatal Disorders for the MRCOG and Beyond *by Andrew Thomson and Iaň Greer*

Fetal Medicine for the MRCOG and Beyond, second edition *by Alan Cameron, Janet Brennand, Lena Crichton and Janice Gibson*

Gynaecological and Obstetric Pathology for the MRCOG and Beyond, second edition *edited by Michael Wells, C Hilary Buckley and Harold Foc, with a chapter on Cervical Cytology by John Smith*

Gynaecological Oncology for the MRCOG and Beyond, second edition *edited by Nigel Acheson and David Luesley*

Gynaecological Urology for the MRCOG and Beyond *by Simon Jackson, Meghana Pandit and Alexandra Blackwell*

Haemorrhage and Thrombosis for the MRCOG and Beyond *edited by Anne Harper*

Management of Infertility for the MRCOG and Beyond *edited by Siladitya Bhattacharya and Mark Hamilton*

Medical Genetics for the MRCOG and Beyond *by Michael Connor*

Menopause for the MRCOG and Beyond, second edition *by Margaret Rees*

Menstrual Problems for the MRCOG *by Mary Ann Lumsden, Jane Norman and Hilary Critchley*

Neonatology for the MRCOG *by Peter Dear and Simon Newell*

Paediatric and Adolescent Gynaecology for the MRCOG and Beyond, second edition *by Anne Garden, Mary Hernan and Joanne Topping*

Psychological Disorders in Obstetrics and Gynaecology for the MRCOG and Beyond, second edition *by Khaled MK Ismail, Ilana Crome and PM Shaughn O'Brien*

Reproductive Endocrinology for the MRCOG and Beyond, second edition *edited by Adam Balen*

The MRCOG: A Guide to the Examination, third edition *edited by William L Ledger and Michael G Murphy*

Intrapartum Care for the MRCOG and Beyond

Second edition

Thomas F Baskett MB, BCh, BAO (The Queen's University of Belfast), FRCS(C), FRCS(Ed), FRCOG, FACOG
Professor, Department of Obstetrics and Gynaecology, Dalhousie University, Halifax, Nova Scotia, Canada

Sabaratnam Arulkumaran MB, BS (University of Ceylon), MD, PhD, FRCS(Ed), FRCOG, FACOG, HonFCOG (SA)
Professor and Head, Department of Obstetrics and Gynaecology, St George's University Medical School, London, UK

With a chapter on neonatal resuscitation
By Gareth J Richards MB, BS, MRCPCH
Consultant Neonatologist, St George's Healthcare NHS Trust, London, UK

And a chapter on perinatal loss
By Austin Ugwumadu MB, BS, PhD, FRCOG
Consultant Obstetrician and Gynaecologist, St George's Healthcare NHS Trust, London, UK
and
Melanie O'Byrne RGN, RM
Specialist Bereavement Midwife, St George's Healthcare NHS Trust, London, UK

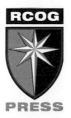

RCOG

PRESS

A machine-readable catalogue record for this publication is available from the British Library [www.bl.uk/catalogue/listings.html]

ISBN 978-1-906985-40-0

Published by the **RCOG Press** at the
Royal College of Obstetricians and Gynaecologists
27 Sussex Place, Regent's Park
London NW1 4RG

Registered Charity No. 213280

Line drawings by Oxford Designers and Illustrators © RCOG
Cover image © Bsip Bajande/Science Photo Library

RCOG Press Editor: Claire Dunn
Index: Cath Topliff
Design & typesetting: FiSH Books, London
Printed by Latimer Trend & Co. Ltd, Estover Road, Plymouth PL6 7PL

Contents

Preface

While maternal and perinatal mortality rates are low in most developed countries, there remain a significant number of ideally preventable deaths in both categories. Furthermore, much of the focus of clinical services is now directed towards preventing the more common severe maternal and neonatal morbidities – the so-called 'near miss' category.

As most of the adverse outcomes are related to labour and delivery, the labour ward is the front line of these endeavours. Caring for women in childbirth is one of the most rewarding aspects of our specialty, but it comes with the need to make rapid decisions under duress and the increasing spectre of litigation. There is a fine clinical balance required from midwives and obstetricians to provide the vigilant care necessary to prevent and manage the relatively rare adverse events during labour, and yet support the wishes of the woman who wants minimal interference.

We have added six new chapters to this second edition of *Intrapartum Care for the MRCOG and Beyond*: improving intrapartum care, lower genital tract trauma, emergency obstetric hysterectomy, acute uterine inversion, disseminated intravascular coagulation and acute tocolysis. We feel that these topics have increasing importance and warrant separate consideration. Each chapter contains limited references, but readers are encouraged to consult the *Pregnancy and Childbirth Module of the Cochrane Database of Systematic Reviews* as well as national and College guidelines.

We have not tried to write each chapter as a detailed review article, although we have incorporated evidence-based medicine and national guidelines where they exist. Our aim has been to produce a concise and pragmatic approach to intrapartum care based on our combined experience on the labour ward over the past 40 years.

Thomas F Baskett and Sabaratnam Arulkumaran

Abbreviations

A B C D	airway, breathing, circulation, drugs
AFE	amniotic fluid embolism
bpm	beats per minute
CTG	cardiotogography
DIC	disseminated intravascular coagulation
ECG	electrocardiogram
EFM	electronic fetal monitoring
ETT	endotracheal tube
FBS	fetal scalp blood sampling
FDP	fibrin degradation products
FHR	fetal heart rate
GBS	group B streptococcus
HELLP syndrome	haemolysis, elevated liver enzymes, low platelets
HIE	hypoxic ischaemic encephalopathy
HIV	human immunodeficiency virus
IV	intravenous
NICE	National Institute for Health and Clinical Excellence
PEEP	positive end-expiratory pressure
PPH	postpartum haemorrhage
PPROM	preterm prelabour rupture of membranes
RCOG	Royal College of Obstetricians and Gynaecologists
RhD	rhesus D
SpO_2	saturation of peripheral oxygen
term PROM	term prelabour rupture of membranes
WHO	World Health Organization

1 Improving intrapartum care

Every mother and her family look forward to normal pregnancy, labour and delivery with a healthy outcome for mother and newborn. The prime responsibility of the caregivers is to ensure this safe outcome and emotional satisfaction in the physiological process of birth.

Broadly speaking, there are four categories of pregnancy:

- the majority of women have a normal pregnancy with spontaneous onset of labour culminating in a normal vaginal delivery
- some women have pre-existing medical conditions that may influence the outcome of pregnancy, such as diabetes, chronic hypertension and obesity
- some women develop obstetric disorders during pregnancy that may have an impact on the pregnancy, labour and delivery, such as pre-eclampsia and obstetric haemorrhage
- in a small number of women, social and psychological factors can have an impact on the progress of pregnancy, labour and delivery.

It is the duty of midwives and obstetricians to provide appropriate care to accommodate the above circumstances.

Surveys in the UK suggest that 90% or more of mothers are satisfied, or more than satisfied, with the care given in pregnancy and labour. The UK has a maternal mortality rate of about 11/100 000 births, while the perinatal mortality rate is about 10/1000; these rates are not low compared with some developed countries and are relatively static. However, the Eighth Report on Confidential Enquiries into Maternal Deaths in the United Kingdom[1] suggests that 50–70% of maternal deaths are associated with substandard care. Adhering to the recommendations of *Safer Childbirth: Minimum Standards for the Organisation and Delivery of Care in Labour*,[2] produced by the Royal College of Anaesthetists, the Royal College of Midwives, the Royal College of Obstetricians and Gynaecologists and the Royal College of Paediatrics and Child Health, should help improve the safety and quality of care given to the mother.

Clinical governance

Clinical governance is a mechanism that enables regular monitoring of clinical care and allows lessons to be learned from clinical outcomes that may help to improve the safety and quality of the care provided. Clinical outcome is dependent on achieving the best performance in the seven essential elements that constitute clinical governance:[3]

- adequate capacity in terms of space, beds, equipment and medications
- adequate numbers of qualified and competent personnel
- evidence-based guidelines
- multiprofessional education and training
- audit of clinical outcome and adherence to guidelines
- risk incident monitoring and management
- promptly addressing and resolving complaints.

Each of these is considered below.

CAPACITY

For a hospital and labour ward to function effectively, there should be an adequate number of beds, necessary operating theatres and recovery rooms and an area for high-dependency care. There should be the equipment needed to provide both routine and emergency care. Women should have a waiting area so that they can rest with their partner and their family before they are taken to the labour room. The labour room should have facilities to allow the partner to stay and provide emotional support to the woman during labour. There should be additional resources to provide women with nutrition. Ideally, there should be attached shower and toilet facilities.

STAFF

There needs to be adequate qualified staff at all levels to look after women in labour: consultant obstetrician, registrars, midwives, anaesthetists and paediatricians. In the UK, the recommended norm is to have one midwife for every 28 deliveries. However, in the current financial climate this may not be feasible and is not achieved by many trusts. The *Safer Childbirth*[2] document provides information on optimal staffing levels for obstetricians, midwives, anaesthetists, paediatricians and midwifery assistants. Table 1.1 provides information regarding recommended obstetric staffing levels based on the size of the maternity unit.

Table 1.1 Recommended obstetric staffing targets based on the number of deliveries

Category	Births/year	Consultant presence (year of adoption) 60 hours	98 hours	168 hours	Specialty trainees (n)
A	<2500	Adequate hours based on local needs			1
B	2500–4000	2009	–	–	2
C1	4000–5000	2008	2009	–	3
C2	5000–6000	Immediate	2008	2010	3
C3	>6000	Immediate	Immediate if possible	2008	3

The staff should be competent in terms of knowledge, skills, attitude and behaviour. Assessment of these factors forms the basis for revalidation of obstetricians every 5 years.[4]

To ensure the best consultant care in critical situations, the RCOG has published Good Practice guidance on *The Responsibility of the Consultant On-call*.[5] The box below shows the recommendations for consultant attendance with the woman and the circumstances when a competent senior registrar can be allowed to provide the care.

RESPONSIBILITY OF THE CONSULTANT ON CALL

Consultant to attend in person:

- Eclampsia
- Maternal collapse (e.g. massive abruption, septic shock)
- Caesarean section for major placenta praevia
- Postpartum haemorrhage over 1.5 l, where the woman is continuing to bleed and massive postpartum haemorrhage protocol has been activated
- Return to operating theatre for laparotomy
- When requested

Consultant to be present unless the specialty trainee is certified to be competent:

- Vaginal breech delivery
- Trial of instrumental vaginal delivery
- Caesarean section at full dilatation
- Caesarean section in a woman whose body mass index is over 40
- Caesarean section at less than 32 weeks of gestation

EVIDENCE-BASED GUIDELINES

Evidence-based guidelines should be available in the labour ward in an electronic format via the intranet and as hard copies in files so that caregivers can easily refer to them to formulate the appropriate management plan for each case. All new staff should be given the information and time to become familiar with the guidelines. The availability of local guidelines based on National Institute for Health and Clinical Excellence guidance (http://guidance.nice.org.uk/Topic/GynaecologyPregnancy Birth) and RCOG Green-top Guidelines (www.rcog.org.uk/guidelines) facilitates multiprofessional working.

EDUCATION AND TRAINING

The presence of guidelines is not sufficient for good clinical outcome. There should be regular multiprofessional education and training so that each profession understands its roles and responsibilities. The Clinical Negligence Scheme for Trusts (www.cnst.org.uk) has promoted multiprofessional learning in the same classroom and practising skills and drills as a team so that, should an emergency arise, there will be no conflict regarding management. Educational training on certain topics can be provided by electronic means, such as the knowledge related to interpretation of cardiotocographs. Audits must be in place to monitor whether practice follows the guidelines.

AUDITS

Each year, a certain number of guidelines should be selected and appropriate audit performed over a short period of time to identify any deficiencies and the reasons behind them. The staff should ascertain problem areas of poor clinical outcome and select these topics for audit. Setting a 'standard' that is to be achieved based on national data is essential before commencing the audit, such as '100% of those at risk should receive prophylaxis for thromboembolism'. The audit should be based on the SMART principle: Specific, Measurable, Achievable, Relevant, Theoretically sound.

Based on the findings, the guidelines may need to be modified or actions taken to achieve better compliance by the staff in following the guidelines.

RISK MANAGEMENT

Risk management is an important process involving the identification of risk incidents, thereby reducing the chance of a poor outcome. Once a risk incident is identified, it is analysed (root-cause analysis) to evaluate the deficiencies that led to the poor outcome and to provide recommendations to prevent such a risk incident recurring. There may be some cost to improve the facilities or training to prevent such recurrences. Multiprofessional training, adequate staff, guidelines, audit and risk management should improve women's safety.

Risks are identified by incident reporting. Staff should be educated and encouraged to report such incidents. The box below contains the trigger list suggested by the RCOG's Clinical Governance Advice No. 2: *Improving Patient Safety: Risk Management for Maternity and Gynaecology.*[6]

TRIGGER LIST FOR INCIDENT REPORTING IN MATERNITY[6]

Maternal	Fetal	Organisational incidents
• Maternal death	• Stillbirth > 500g	• Unavailability of health records
• Undiagnosed breech	• Neonatal death	
• Shoulder dystocia	• Agpar score < 7 at 5 minutes	• Delay in responding to call for assistance
• Blood loss > 1500ml		
• Return to operating theatre	• Birth trauma	• Unplanned home birth
	• Fetal laceration at caesarean section	
• Eclampsia		• Faulty equipment
• Hysterectomy/ laparotomy	• Cord pH < 7.05/ venous blood pH < 7.1	• Conflict over case management
• Anaesthetic complication		• Potential user complaint
	• Neonatal seizures	
• Admission to intensive care unit	• Term baby admitted to neonatal unit	• Medication error
		• Retained swab/ instrument
• Venous thromboembolism	• Undiagnosed fetal anomaly	
		• Hospital-acquired infection
• Third- and fourth-degree tears		
		• Violation of local protocol
• Unsuccessful forceps/ventouse delivery		
• Uterine rupture		
• Readmission of mother		

COMPLAINTS AND COMMUNICATION

Complaints should be categorised according to whether they are a result of system error, clinical error or attitude and communication. There should be zero tolerance for complaints related to attitude and communication in a sensitive environment like the labour ward. All staff should remind their colleagues to avoid such incidents and complaints.

Risk incidents and complaints can be reduced by committed, compassionate and competent care. Improving patient handover is a key to avoid clinical errors. The RCOG's Good Practice No. 12: *Improving patient handover*[7] provides useful information on proper handover. There are a number of tools to facilitate effective handover. The most commonly used is SBAR: **S**ituation, **B**ackground, **A**ssessment, **R**ecommendation:

- When we deal with a woman, we should provide the information of her name, location, vital signs and any specific concerns.

- This should be followed by the woman's background, including the date of admission, diagnosis, medication, test results and information needed to make a proper assessment and diagnosis.

- Assessment involves critical evaluation of the situation based on the background provided.

- The clinician should make a recommendation, which should be in the form of a management plan.

- This approach provides for effective communication at handover and should be used for every woman, especially at staff change-over.

Clinical governance and performance chart (the Maternity Dashboard)

The information on the different elements of clinical governance and clinical performance in a unit can be plotted on a daily, weekly or monthly basis as a 'dashboard' (like that of a car), highlighting areas of concern in amber or red to attract the attention of the clinician and the administrator. The information is useful for the provider (the hospital), for women, for the commissioner of services and for the regulators (such as the Care Quality Commission). This information, captured on one page on a monthly basis, provides guidance as to how things are improving or deteriorating. The green, amber and red boxes for each parameter enable clinicians and administrators to rectify problems in the amber zone before they deteriorate to red. The RCOG provides an example of a Maternity Dashboard in Good Practice No. 7: *Maternity Dashboard: Clinical Performance and Governance Score Card.*[8]

Continuous monitoring of such information ensures that clinicians and management take an interest and work towards a better outcome, and also provides a focus for clinical and administrative teamwork. For example, if the number of admissions to the intensive care unit following postpartum haemorrhage falls and there is a concomitant reduction in postpartum hysterectomy and blood transfusion as the months progress, it suggests better care and teamwork. On the other hand, if the incidence of anal sphincter damage increases, one needs to question why this is so and organise workshops at suitable times to train staff in the prevention and correct repair of anal sphincter injury.

Conclusion

The definition of safe patient care is good clinical outcome without adverse incident caused by the treatment given. Quality is built on safety when there is mental and emotional wellbeing at the end of care; this is of paramount importance in maternity care and may determine whether the woman wants to embark upon another pregnancy.

Healthcare professionals need to practise in the best possible way, adhering to evidence-based guidelines and standards of expected care.[2,5,7–9] To provide the best care, we should acquire knowledge and technical expertise and improve teamwork through multidisciplinary training in skills and drills. Adherence to guidelines needs to be checked by regular audits. Root-cause analysis of risk incidents and complaints and appropriate recommendations are essential for us to continually improve the care given. As professionals, we should act in the best interests of women to provide competent and compassionate care.

References

1. Centre for Maternal and Child Enquiries. Saving Mothers' Lives: reviewing maternal deaths to make motherhood safer: 2006–08. The Eighth Report on Confidential Enquiries into Maternal Deaths in the United Kingdom. *BJOG* 2011;118 Suppl 1:1–203.
2. Royal College of Anaesthetists, Royal College of Midwives, Royal College of Obstetricians and Gynaecologists, Royal College of Paediatrics and Child Health. *Safer Childbirth: Minimum Standards for the Organisation and Delivery of Care in Labour*. London: RCOG Press; 2007 [http://www.rcog.org.uk/womens-health/clinical-guidance/safer-childbirth-minimum-standards-organisation-and-delivery-care-la].
3. Arulkumaran S. Clinical governance and standards in UK maternity care to improve quality and safety. *Midwifery* 2010;26:485–7.
4. NHS Professionals, General Medical Council. GMC and NHS Professionals Revalidation Project. Final Report: August 2009. London: GMC; 2009 [http://www.gmc-uk.org/doctors/licensing/revalidation_system_readiness_projects.asp].
5. Royal College of Obstetricians and Gynaecologists. *Responsibility of Consultant On-call*. Good Practice Guideline No. 8. London: RCOG; 2009 [http://www.rcog.org.uk/responsibility-of-consultant-on-call].
6. Royal College of Obstetricians and Gynaecologists. *Improving Patient Safety: Risk Management for Maternity and Gynaecology*. Clinical Governance Advice

No. 2. London: RCOG; 2009 [http://www.rcog.org.uk/improving-patient-safety-risk-management-maternity-and-gynaecology].

7. Royal College of Obstetricians and Gynaecologists. *Improving patient handover*. Good Practice No. 12. London: RCOG; 2010 [http://www.rcog.org.uk/womens-health/clinical-guidance/improving-patient-handover-good-practice-no-12].

8. Royal College of Obstetricians and Gynaecologists. *Maternity Dashboard: Clinical Performance and Governance Score Card*. Good Practice No. 7. London: RCOG; 2008 [http://www.rcog.org.uk/womens-health/clinical-guidance/maternity-dashboard-clinical-performance-and-governance-score-card].

9. Royal College of Anaesthetists, Royal College of Midwives, Royal College of Obstetricians and Gynaecologists, Royal College of Paediatrics and Child Health. *Standards for Maternity Care. Report of a Working Party*. London: RCOG Press; 2008 [http://www.rcog.org.uk/womens-health/clinical-guidance/standards-maternity-care].

2 First stage of labour

Labour and delivery are sentinel events in a woman's life and her experience, good or bad, may have a profound effect on her attitude to her infant, her husband and the prospect of future pregnancy. In this context, the outcome of a woman's first labour and delivery is paramount. As O'Driscoll stated, 'A woman who has had a happy first experience is unlikely to suffer much apprehension about a later birth, whereas a woman who has had an unhappy first experience is likely to be terrified at the prospect of a repeat performance. These fears can have grave consequences outside the narrow confines of obstetrics; they can haunt a woman for the rest of her life and affect her attitude to her husband and also possibly to her child.'[1]

Primigravid labour is usually longer and more painful than subsequent labours; if the woman can be guided through her first labour to a safe vaginal delivery with physical and emotional security, her future obstetric experience is likely to be uncomplicated.[2]

The first stage of labour starts with the onset of regular painful uterine contractions that lead to the progressive effacement and dilatation of the cervix, ending when the cervix has reached full dilatation.

Diagnosis of labour

Establishing the diagnosis of labour is the most basic and essential aspect of labour-ward management.[1,3] In no other branch of clinical medicine do we expect the patient to make a diagnosis upon which will be based all future management. Happily, most women at term who present themselves to hospital believing they are in labour are correct. A presumed diagnosis of labour is based upon the onset of regular and painful contractions which are of increasing frequency and severity. This is often associated with a blood-stained mucous 'show' and, less often, rupture of the membranes. However, for the diagnosis of labour to be clearly established, these symptoms and signs have to be associated with significant change in effacement and dilatation of the cervix. The most important aspect, indeed the sine qua non, is effacement of the cervix; provided this has occurred, the diagnosis is confirmed. Most women believing themselves to be in labour can have this diagnosis confirmed and a smaller number with a completely uneffaced cervix can be assured that they are not in labour. There remains a group, accounting for about 10–15% of women who believe themselves to be in labour, in whom neither the woman nor the attendant can confirm whether or not they are in progressive labour. In such cases the woman should be told this and be observed over the next 2–6 hours, when repeat assessment of the cervix should lead to a firm diagnosis. This period of observation should be carried out away from the active labour ward if at all possible. If an incorrect diagnosis of labour is made, a series of inappropriate interventions (amniotomy, oxytocin augmentation, operative delivery) may ensue over a long and demoralising period.[1,3]

Assessment of labour

There are three main components in the assessment and management of the first stage of labour:

- progress of labour
- condition of the mother
- condition of the fetus.

In this chapter the fetus is discussed at term in cephalic presentation.

PROGRESS OF LABOUR

Uterine contractions are recorded by their frequency, duration and strength (Figure 2.1). The state of the cervix is recorded in terms of its effacement and dilatation. In addition, other features such as anterior or mid-position of the cervix in early labour, along with a soft and distensible consistency as labour progresses, are favourable signs. On the other hand, posterior position of the cervix in early labour and a thickened and oedematous consistency as labour progresses are less favourable signs.

The main function of uterine contractions in the first stage of labour is cervical effacement and dilatation. To a lesser degree there is descent of the presenting part, although the majority of descent occurs in the second stage of labour.

CHARTING THE PROGRESS OF LABOUR

Friedman developed the basis for scientific study of the progress of labour by graphically depicting the rate of cervical dilatation against time.[4] Friedman's cervicogram forms the basis of the modern partogram and incorporates aspects of the progress of labour along with the

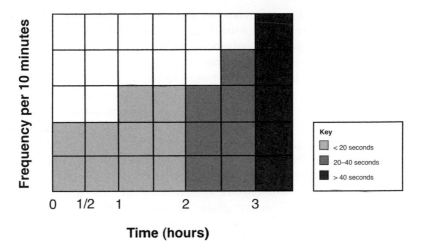

Time (hours)

Figure 2.1 Quantification of uterine contractions by clinical palpation; frequency per 10 minutes is recorded by shading the equivalent number of boxes; the type of shading indicates the duration of each contraction

condition of the mother and the fetus in a chronological manner on one page. The parameters of labour progress include:

- frequency and duration of uterine contractions
- cervical effacement and dilatation
- descent, caput and moulding of the presenting part.

The maternal condition is recorded by temperature, pulse, blood pressure and drugs administered. The fetal condition is recorded by the colour and quantity of amniotic fluid passed and the fetal heart rate. This pictorial documentation of labour ensures a systematic and logical appraisal which facilitates early recognition of poor progress. Nomograms of cervical dilatation confirm that different ethnic groups have similar rates of cervical dilatation and uterine activity in spontaneous labour. The rate of cervical dilatation has two phases:

- a slow, so-called latent phase during which the cervix shortens from about 3 cm in length to less than 0.5 cm (effacement) and dilates to 3 cm
- a faster active phase, when the cervix dilates from 3 cm to full dilatation.

To identify those at risk of prolonged labour, a line of acceptable progress known as the 'alert line' is drawn on the partogram. If the rate of cervical dilatation crosses to the right of the alert line, progress is deemed unsatisfactory. The line of acceptable progress can be based on the mean, median or slowest tenth percentile rate of cervical dilatation in women who progress without intervention and deliver normally. Intervention is thought to be necessary if the rate of progress cuts the 'action line', which is drawn parallel and 1–4 hours to the right of the alert line.[5,6] Thus, depending on which of the above criteria is applied, the proportion of labours deemed to have unsatisfactory progress can vary from 5% to 50%. Each unit will develop its own guidelines that define non-progressive labour, but the principle of partographic depiction of labour should be universally applied. This approach has been endorsed by the World Health Organization (Figure 2.2).[7] The latent phase of labour may last up to 8 hours in nulliparous women and up to 6 hours in multiparous women. In the active phase of labour both nulliparous and multiparous women dilate at a rate of least 1 cm/hour, with the multiparous woman usually dilating much more rapidly.

MATERNAL CONDITION

Upon admission to the labour floor, the antenatal chart is reviewed and an abbreviated history and physical examination performed. This will include temperature, pulse, blood pressure, abdominal palpation, fetal heart auscultation and urinalysis. Depending on the woman's history of uterine contractions, show and rupture of membranes, a vaginal examination may be performed to confirm the diagnosis of labour, or this may be postponed until later. If the diagnosis of labour is confirmed, this should be reviewed with the woman and an optimistic approach conveyed about forthcoming events. If the woman is in early labour, she may wish to have fluids and a light snack. If she is established in active labour, sips of water, ice chips and sucking hard sweets are more appropriate.

If the pregnancy is low risk and it is likely that delivery will occur within 6–8 hours, an intravenous infusion is not necessary. However, if the mother requires epidural anaesthesia or becomes dehydrated, or should labour be prolonged or high risk, an intravenous infusion of crystalloids or dextrose/saline should be established.

When possible, the woman should be up and walking during the first stage of labour. She should be encouraged to assume whatever position she finds most comfortable, which is usually sitting, reclining or the lateral semi-recumbent position.

No woman in labour should be left alone. While some partners are helpful during labour, they cannot replace a knowledgeable nurse or midwife. Each hospital will develop its own guidelines for the attendance of companions and family members in labour, but the roles of such

PARTOGRAPH

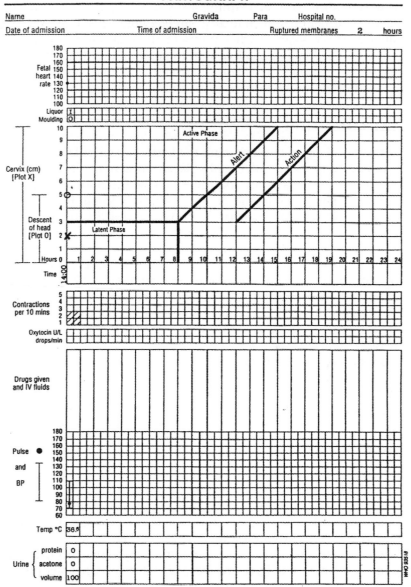

Figure 2.2 World Health Organization partograph showing alert and action lines in the latent and active phases of labour; cervical dilatation, descent of head, fetal parameters (fetal heart rate, colour of liquor, caput and moulding) and maternal parameters (pulse, blood pressure, results of urine tests and drugs used) can be entered

companions with regard to the nursing and medical staff should be clearly established.

Explanation of progress and any interventions should be carefully outlined to the woman and her partner. Although there is enormous pressure on nursing and medical staff to chart all events for audit and medico-legal purposes, a balance between this and common sense, clinical care and communication must be achieved.

FETAL CONDITION

Generally speaking, in low-risk cases the fetus that enters labour in good condition is unlikely to suffer asphyxia during a normally progressive labour. Thus, if the fetal heart at the start of labour is normal, there is no meconium staining and the subsequent progress of labour is normal, the outlook for delivery of a normal, well-oxygenated infant is excellent. Auscultation of the fetal heart rate for at least 1 minute immediately after a contraction every 15 minutes in the first stage of labour is adequate. If the pregnancy is high risk, there is any abnormality of the fetal heart rate or meconium staining of the amniotic fluid, continuous electronic fetal heart rate monitoring is advisable. Various options can be made available: if auscultation every 15 minutes is not feasible, or at the request of the woman, a compromise is to have a 10–20-minute admission screening test with external electronic fetal heart rate monitoring.[8] If the results of this test are completely normal and the amniotic fluid is clear, intermittent auscultation every 15 minutes may replace the electronic fetal heart monitor if the woman wishes. The details of fetal surveillance in labour are outlined in chapter 4.

ANALGESIA

Childbirth classes that include education and training in relaxation and breathing techniques help some women in labour. However, the majority, particularly primiparous women, will request additional analgesia.

Randomised trials have shown that continuous support and explanation, not always from a professional midwife or nurse, shortens labour, lessens requirements for analgesia and reduces operative delivery rates.[9]

Systemic narcotic analgesia is most often given using pethidine. The dose ranges from 50 mg to 150 mg intramuscularly. Analgesia is usually given in the first stage of labour and probably has its main benefit in anxious women with painful early labour. It can be given in 25 mg increments intravenously every 3–5 minutes to give rapid relief in a woman in whom pain has been allowed to get out of control. Fentanyl, a highly lipid-soluble synthetic opioid, can be used as an alternative to meperidine, to which it has similar but less pronounced adverse effects.[11] Fentanyl is given as an intravenous dose of 50–100 micrograms or in a patient-controlled intravenous analgesia set-up. There is no evidence that patient-controlled intravenous analgesia provides superior analgesia, but it does reduce the total amount of drug given. Other than a delay in gastric emptying, which may be relevant if subsequent general anaesthesia is required, meperidine and fentanyl have no serious maternal adverse effects in the doses used. The main potential drawback is respiratory depression in the newborn if delivery occurs 1–3 hours after administration to the mother. This can be dealt with by providing assisted ventilation to the infant and administering the narcotic antagonist naloxone in a dose of 0.1 mg/kg by intramuscular injection; alternatively, if the infant requires an endotracheal tube, naloxone can be given by this route (see also chapter 25, page 269).

Inhalation analgesia is simple and safe, but is effective in only a minority of women. The most practical and safest form is a 50% nitrous oxide and 50% oxygen mixture, which comes in a variety of devices for self-administration. There is a latent period between the woman starting inhalation and there being sufficient gas tension in her central nervous system to produce analgesia. This usually takes five to six deep breaths and it is therefore important to help the woman start breathing the gas before she feels the pain of the uterine contraction. This can be achieved by timing, if the contractions are very regular, or by the fact that a uterine contraction is palpable before the woman feels the pain. In general, this method of analgesia can be exhausting and dehydrating if used for too long. Its main benefit is in the woman, usually multiparous, in the late first stage of labour when labour is progressing rapidly and becoming very painful. This will often see the woman through the late first stage and early second stage until she can begin bearing-down efforts.

While skillfully applied narcotic and inhalation analgesia may be adequate for a number of women, particularly multiparous women, many will request epidural analgesia. Details of the administration of epidural analgesia are beyond the scope of this book, but those who have worked in units with and without this service will attest to the enormous humane benefits that this technique of pain relief has brought to labour. Epidural analgesia does not interfere with progress in the first stage of labour but it can have a profound effect in the second stage; this is discussed in chapter 3.

Management of non-progressive labour

CAUSES

It is still reasonable to consider the three Ps – the 'powers', the 'passages' and the 'passenger' – in the causation of non-progressive labour. Often a combination of all three is responsible.

- **Powers**: The most practical clinical approach to the powers is to consider uterine action effective or ineffective depending on whether it causes appropriate dilatation of the cervix.

- **Passages**: The passages are assessed clinically. In the developed world a contracted pelvis is extremely rare, but previous pelvic fractures may be relevant. Soft-tissue obstruction, such as a cervical fibroid, is also rare. X-ray pelvimetry is of no help in the clinical management of non-progressive labour.

- **Passenger**: The passenger may be too large for the pelvis or, more frequently, the fetal head may be deflexed in the occipitotransverse or occipitoposterior position. This deflexion can present as much as 1.5 cm increased diameter to the bony pelvis. Malpresentations such as brow should also be sought. With antenatal care and ultrasound it is rare nowadays for a fetal anomaly such as hydrocephaly to be first discovered during labour.

AUGMENTATION OF LABOUR

Augmentation of the active phase of labour can be carried out by amniotomy and, if this fails, by oxytocin augmentation. The procedure for oxytocin infusion is given in chapter 7, page 78. Once the partogram shows non-progressive labour, the number of women who receive augmentation depends on how quickly one feels this should be instituted. In the Dublin active management of labour protocol, augmentation is started after a 1-hour delay in progress, which occurs in about half of all nulliparous women.[1] If a delay of 2 hours is accepted before instituting augmentation, about 20% will require augmentation. Depending on the staffing in various units and the wishes of the woman, one may allow 1–4 hours before augmentation is instituted; the World Health Organization recommends 4 hours.[7]

The intrapartum care guidelines produced by the National Institute for Health and Clinical Excellence[10] define slow progress as follows:

- cervical dilatation less than 2 cm in 4 hours with no alteration in any other labour progress index; or

- cervical progress less than 2 cm in 6 hours where there may have been changes in other labour progress indices and the membranes have been ruptured for at least 2 hours; or

- cervical progress less than 3 cm in 8 hours where amniotomy has been performed late, but at least 2 hours previously, and where there may have been changes in other labour progress indices.

Other labour progress indices are related to parity, the state of the membranes, descent and rotation of the presenting part and clinical assessment of uterine contractions.

The above definitions were introduced to reduce unnecessary oxytocin augmentation, as the benefits of early augmentation have not been conclusively established. Although there is no 'correct' answer in women with non-progressive labour, the principle of correcting inefficient uterine action with augmentation by amniotomy and oxytocin appears to be sound and is established in clinical practice.

If there is delay in the early part of the active phase, between 3 and 7 cm dilation, it is sometimes called primary dysfunctional labour or protraction disorder. This is often a combination of relative disproportion owing to deflexion of the fetal head and ineffective uterine action. Many of these cases will respond well to augmentation. Secondary arrest of labour after 7 cm dilation may have the same genesis but more often is a result of cephalopelvic disproportion (Figure 2.3). In either event the only influence the obstetrician can bring to bear is to improve uterine action and hope there will be flexion and rotation of the fetal head, which presents a smaller diameter to the pelvis and leads to progressive cervical dilatation and descent of the head.[12] In the second stage of labour, relative cephalopelvic disproportion owing to deflexion of the occipitoposterior position may flex and rotate with the application of appropriate forceps or vacuum traction (see chapter 9).

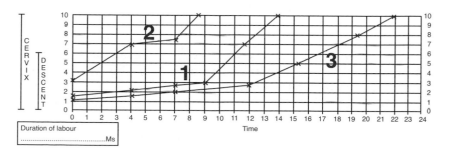

Figure 2.3 Abnormal labour patterns: (1) prolonged latent phase, (2) secondary arrest, (3) prolonged latent phase and primary dysfunctional labour

Non-progressive labour is a very trying event for all concerned. Care during labour should be directed towards sustaining the morale of the woman and her partner, maintaining maternal hydration, providing adequate analgesia and, where possible, correcting the cause of the lack of progress.

References

1. O'Driscoll K, Meagher D, Robson M. *Active Management of Labour (fourth edition)*. London: Mosby; 2003.
2. Mawdsley SW, Baskett TF. Outcome of the next labour in women who had a vaginal delivery in their first pregnancy. *BJOG* 2000;107:932–4.
3. Reuwer P, Bruinse H, Franx A. *Proactive Support of Labor: The Challenge of Normal Childbirth*. Cambridge: Cambridge University Press; 2009.
4. Friedman EA. Primigravid labor: a graphicostatistical analysis. *Obstet Gynecol* 1955;6:567–89.
5. Philpott RH, Castle WM. Cervicographs in the management of labour in primigravidae. I. The alert line for detecting abnormal labour. *J Obstet Gynaecol Br Commonw* 1972;79:592–8.
6. Philpott RH, Castle WM. Cervicographs in the management of labour in primigravidae. II. The action line and treatment of abnormal labour. *J Obstet Gynaecol Br Commonw* 1972;79:599–602.
7. World Health Organization partograph in management of labour. World Health Organization Maternal Health and Safe Motherhood Programme. *Lancet* 1994;343:1399–404.
8. Ingemarsson I, Arulkumaran S, Ingemarssan E, Tambyraja RL, Ratnam SS. Admission test: a screening test for fetal distress in labor. *Obstet Gynecol* 1986;68:800–6.
9. Kennell J, Klaus M, McGrath S, Robertson S, Hinkley C. Continuous emotional support during labor in a US hospital. A randomized controlled trial. *JAMA* 1991;265:2197–201.
10. National Institute for Health and Clinical Excellence. NICE clinical guideline 55: *Intrapartum care. Care of healthy women and their babies during childbirth*. London: NICE; 2007. p. 138–55.
11. Reynolds F. The effects of maternal labour analgesia on the fetus. *Best Pract Res Clin Obstet Gynaecol* 2010;24:289–302.
12. Fitzpatrick M, McQuillan K, O'Herlihy C. Influence of persistent occiput posterior position on delivery outcome. *Obstet Gynecol* 2001;98:1027–31.

3 Second stage of labour

The second stage of labour lasts from full dilatation of the cervix to delivery of the infant. It is the stage when the fetus is most vulnerable, with hypoxia and trauma being the main threats. This was highlighted in the 4th Annual Report of the Confidential Inquiry into Stillbirths and Deaths in Infancy,[1] emphasising the clinical and medico-legal aspects of the second stage of labour.

The second stage has two phases: the first, passive, phase occurs from full dilatation of the cervix until the head descends to the pelvic floor and the second, active, phase starts when bearing-down efforts of the mother begin. Thus, the terms passive and active refer to maternal effort. The two phases may also be referred to as the pelvic and perineal phases. In the multiparous woman the passive phase can be very brief and last only a few minutes. However, in the nulliparous woman the head is often at the level of the ischial spines when full dilatation is reached and more time and uterine action is required to cause descent of the presenting part to the pelvic floor. In this and other aspects of care during labour, it is important to differentiate between the performance of the nulliparous and multiparous woman.

Utero–fetal–pelvic relationships

The relationship between maternal effort, uterine action, the fetal presenting part and the pelvis is dynamic rather than a mechanical set of measurements. The following factors require evaluation and, as in the first stage of labour, can still be usefully considered under the old classification of the three Ps (see box overleaf).

UTERINE WORK

In considering uterine work, it is essential to be aware of the effect of epidural analgesia. In the second stage of normal spontaneous labour there is an increase in the endogenous production of oxytocin, which augments uterine action and aids descent of the presenting part. This physiological increase of oxytocin is blocked by epidural anaesthesia owing to the interruption of Ferguson's reflex.[2] It is therefore often

THE THREE Ps	
Powers	• Uterine • Maternal
Passenger	• Size • Malposition • Malpresentation • Anomaly
Passages	• Bony pelvis • Soft tissues

necessary to start or increase oxytocin augmentation during the second stage of labour when epidural analgesia is in place. Epidural anaesthesia also blunts the maternal bearing-down reflex; this applies to both nulliparous and multiparous women, although with appropriate coaching the multiparous woman can usually apply adequate maternal effort. More sophisticated epidural techniques with selective sensory blocks are an improvement in this regard. An understanding of the effect of epidural analgesia on the second stage of labour and the need to replace the usual physiological increase of oxytocin production can, to some extent, counteract the prolongation of the second stage of labour and need for assisted vaginal delivery with epidural analgesia.[3,4]

MATERNAL EFFORT

Maternal bearing-down effort should not be encouraged until the head has descended to the pelvic floor. This is particularly relevant in the nulliparous woman, in whom full cervical dilatation is often reached when the head is still at the level of the mid-pelvis.[5] At this point, maternal pushing will be unproductive, exhausting and demoralising. There is a limit to how long a woman can push productively in the second stage of labour (usually about 1 hour) and this resource should not be squandered when the head is at the level of the mid-pelvis. The traditional 'coached' method of pushing is to encourage the woman to take a deep breath and push against a closed glottis (Valsalva manoeuvre) for as long as she can hold her breath: usually about 8–10 seconds. This type of coached pushing is associated with a reduction in the duration of the second stage of labour;[6] however, it is also associated with a rise in maternal intrathoracic pressure and decreased venous return and cardiac output, which can result in reduced uteroplacental circulation. As a result, there are more abnormalities of the fetal heart rate, lower cord pH and lower Apgar scores with this technique. If the woman is not coached, she will often push for 3–5 seconds every 10 seconds or so during the contraction. Furthermore, she will tend not to use the full Valsalva manoeuvre. The net result is a slightly longer second stage of labour but less disruption to the uteroplacental circulation and therefore better fetal oxygenation.[7]

MATERNAL POSITION

Throughout the ages women have adopted, or been advised to adopt, just about every position imaginable in the second stage of labour. The general principles of common sense and the woman's own choice should guide matters. The worst position is supine, which is mechanically illogical and also associated with potential aortocaval compression, which leads to more fetal heart rate abnormalities and lower Apgar scores.[8] In general, upright positions are more comfortable and logical. Kneeling, squatting, sitting and all-fours positions all have their advocates.[9] Some of these positions are quite hard to maintain for long periods of time. It is probably advantageous for the woman to change her position during the second stage of labour. Many will choose the semi-recumbent position alternating with squatting, kneeling or the lateral position.

FETAL HEAD

The size of the fetus may be such that it is too large to pass through the woman's pelvis. Malposition of the fetal head, usually occipitoposterior, presents a larger diameter to the pelvis; this is compounded if the head is deflexed as well as occipitoposterior. Malpresentations, such as brow, and fetal anomalies, such as hydrocephaly, are less common causes of cephalopelvic disproportion.

BONY PELVIS

Assessment of the bony pelvis during the pelvic examination, while subjective, is a worthwhile exercise and, with experience, useful information can be obtained. Each attendant on the labour floor should measure their own fingers and fist, which will enable them to assess some of the following aspects of the bony pelvis:

- The diagonal conjugate from the sacral promontory to the inner aspect of the symphysis should measure at least 12 cm.
- The sacrum should be nicely curved with the lower end not too prominent anteriorly.

- The pelvic side walls should be parallel rather than convergent.
- The prominence of the ischial spines should be noted and the sacro-spinous ligaments should be palpated and accept at least two fingers (4 cm).
- The subpubic arch should not be unduly narrowed (should accommo-date two fingers) and the inter-tuberous diameter should be at least 10 cm (should accommodate four knuckles).

It is recognised that many of the above measurements are rather subjective and that male and female hands vary in size, but with practice individuals can gain valuable clinical experience about the bony fetal–pelvic relationships in labour.

ASSESSMENT OF PROGRESS

Accurate assessment of the level of the fetal head in the pelvis is the essential component of progress in the second stage. The following elements should be assessed.

Position of the fetal head

The position of the fetal head may be occipitoanterior (presenting diameter: suboccipitobregmatic 9.5 cm), which is the most favourable, or occipitotransverse or occipitoposterior. The latter two positions tend to be associated with varying degrees of deflexion, which presents a larger diameter of the fetal head to the bony pelvis: up to 11.5 cm with occipitofrontal deflexion.

Asynclitism

It is common to have a degree of asynclitism, such that one parietal bone presents more prominently than the other with the head in the transverse position as it enters the pelvis. Anterior asynclitism, with more of the parietal bone felt in the anterior half of the pelvis and the sagittal suture towards the posterior half of the pelvis, is physiological, but posterior asynclitism is unfavourable and may indicate disproportion (Figure 3.1).

Caput

Caput is a rather subjective assessment of the amount of oedema in the scalp soft tissues. Caput is rated as +, ++ or +++.

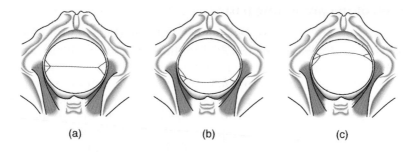

(a)   (b)   (c)

Figure 3.1 Synclitism and asynclitism (left occiput transverse position)

(a)   Normal synclitism: both parietal bones present equally
(b)   Anterior asynclitism: the anterior parietal bone presents
(c)   Posterior asynclitism: the posterior parietal bone presents

Moulding

Moulding (Figure 3.2) may be classified as follows:

- none = bones normally separated
- + = bones touching
- ++ = bones overlapping but easily reduced with digital pressure
- +++ = bones overlapping and not reducible with digital pressure.

The finding of + and ++ degrees of moulding is quite compatible with normal progress and vaginal delivery, whereas +++, along with failure to descend, is usually a sign of cephalopelvic disproportion.

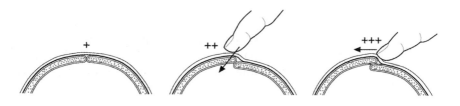

Figure 3.2 Degrees of moulding

+   Parietal bones touching but not overlapping
++   Parietal bones overlap but easily reduced with digital pressure
+++ Parietal bones overlap and not reducible with digital pressure

Station of the presenting part

The station of the presenting part is defined as the level of the lowest part of the fetal bony skull in relation to the ischial spines. With varying degrees of caput and moulding it can be very difficult to assess the true level of the bony part in relation to the ischial spines by vaginal examination alone. Thus, vaginal assessment of the descent of the fetal head measured in centimetres above or below the ischial spines is combined with abdominal assessment of the level of the fetal head in fifths above the pelvic brim (Figure 3.3), with one-fifth being roughly equal to one finger-breadth above the pubic symphysis.[10] A head that is one-fifth palpable above the pelvic brim will be just at the ischial spines. A head that is at spines +1 cm to +2 cm will not be palpable at the pelvic brim. The difference between these two levels can be crucial in the decision for or against assisted vaginal delivery (see chapter 9, page 103).

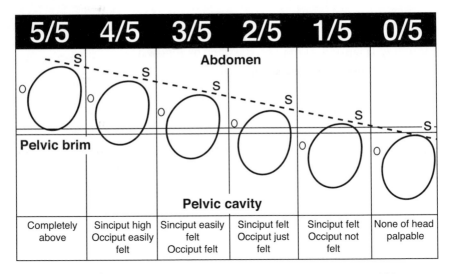

5/5	4/5	3/5	2/5	1/5	0/5
Completely above	Sinciput high Occiput easily felt	Sinciput easily felt Occiput felt	Sinciput felt Occiput just felt	Sinciput felt Occiput not felt	None of head palpable

Figure 3.3 Clinical estimation of the descent of the fetal head in fifths palpable above the pelvic brim; O = occiput; S = sinciput

DURATION

In most women there is clear clinical progress in the second stage of labour, with descent of the head to the pelvic floor, maternal bearing-down effort, lengthening of the perineum with contractions and gradual dilatation of the anus so that the anterior mucosa of the anal canal is seen, showing that the head is low in the pelvis.

In the normally progressive second stage of labour without epidural analgesia, most multiparous women will be delivered within 30 minutes and nulliparous women within 60 minutes. There are, however, many exceptions to this: duration is influenced by parity, fetal weight, malposition of the fetal head (deflexed occipitotransverse and occipito-posterior), maternal effort, effectiveness of uterine contractions and epidural analgesia. Thus, no specific time limit is put on the duration of the second stage of labour provided that the maternal and fetal condition are satisfactory.

While there should be no set time limit, maternal and perinatal morbidity have been shown to rise as the duration of the second stage of labour increases.[11] Thus, guidelines have been established to assess progress, or lack thereof, so that appropriate intervention can be considered.[12] The second stage of labour is considered prolonged in nulliparous women after 2 hours without regional anaesthesia and 3 hours with regional anaesthesia; the corresponding figures for multiparous women are 1 hour and 2 hours, respectively.[12] There is arrest of progress in the second stage of labour if there is no descent of the fetal head after 30 minutes in multiparous women and 60 minutes in nulliparous women. Protracted progress is less than 2 cm descent per hour in multiparous women and less than 1 cm descent per hour in nulliparous women. Most cases of inadequate progress in the second stage of labour are in nulliparous women.

These factors are considered in detail in chapter 9, page 100.

FETAL HEART RATE CHANGES

In normal labour, fetal heart rate can be monitored adequately by auscultation after each contraction in the second stage of labour. If there is doubt, and in high-risk pregnancies, continuous fetal heart rate monitoring should be carried out because this is the time of maximal hypoxic stress. Details of fetal assessment in labour are provided in chapter 4. In essence, it is common to see early decelerations in the fetal heart rate in the second stage of labour as a result of head compression. If there are no other abnormalities, these decelerations are regarded as physiological. Mild to moderate variable decelerations are also common in the second stage of labour but, provided the recovery is rapid and the baseline variability normal, these need not be a reason for intervention.

ANALGESIA

Analgesia during the second stage of labour may just be an extension of epidural analgesia from the first stage of labour, in which case the previous comments about oxytocin augmentation of the second stage may be relevant. If the woman has not required epidural analgesia, inhalation analgesia may be effective, particularly for the multiparous woman with a short second stage of labour. Skilful application of this technique is necessary if it is to be beneficial, as outlined in chapter 2, page 15.

If episiotomy is deemed necessary, infiltration of the perineum with local anaesthesia is appropriate. Analgesic techniques for assisted vaginal delivery are considered in chapter 9, page 104.

Care of the perineum and lower genital tract trauma is covered in chapter 6.

While there is an increasing amount of evidence-based data on the second stage of labour, much of the management is based on the individual clinician's skill and judgement. The second stage of labour is the most dramatic stage of pregnancy during which the very essence of the art of midwifery and obstetrics is brought to bear. It is easy for the accoucheur to get caught up in the drama and one therefore has to remember the essential elements – the condition of the mother and the fetus – so that hasty, ill-considered decisions are not taken that might jeopardise the safety of either.

References

1. Confidential Enquiry into Stillbirths and Deaths in Infancy. *4th Annual Report 1995*. London: Maternal and Child Health Research Consortium; 1997.
2. Goodfellow CF, Hull MG, Swaab DF, Dogterom J, Buijs RM. Oxytocin deficiency at delivery with epidural analgesia. *Br J Obstet Gynaecol* 1983;90:14–9.
3. Bates RG, Helm CW, Duncan A, Edmonds DK. Uterine activity in the second stage of labour and the effect of epidural analgesia. *Br J Obstet Gynaecol* 1985;92:1246–50.
4. Saunders N, Spiby H, Gilbert L, Fraser RB, Hall JM, Mutton PM, et al. Oxytocin infusion during second stage of labour in primiparous women using epidural analgesia: a randomised double blind placebo controlled trial. *BMJ* 1989;299:1423–6.
5. Vause S, Congdon HM, Thornton JG. Immediate and delayed pushing in the second stage of labour for nulliparous women with epidural analgesia: a randomised controlled trial. *Br J Obstet Gynaecol* 1998;105:186–8.
6. Bloom SL, Casey BM, Schaffer JI, McIntire DD, Leveno KJ. A randomized trial of coached versus uncoached maternal pushing during the second stage of labor. *Am J Obstet Gynecol* 2006;194:10–13.
7. Hansen SL, Clark SL, Foster JC. Active pushing versus passive fetal descent in the second stage of labor: a randomized controlled trial. *Obstet Gynecol* 2002;99:29–34.

8. de Jong PR, Johanson RB, Baxen P, Adrians PD, van der Westhuisen S, Jones PW. Randomised trial comparing the upright and supine positions for the second stage of labour. *Br J Obstet Gynaecol* 1997;104:567–71.

9. Ragnar I, Altman D, Tydén T, Olsson SE. Comparison of the maternal experience and duration of labour in two upright delivery positions – a randomised controlled trial. *BJOG* 2006;113:165–70.

10. Notelovitz M. Graphic records in labour. *Br Med J* 1973;1:50.

11. Allen VM, Baskett TF, O'Connell CM, McKeen D, Allen AC. Maternal and perinatal outcomes with increasing duration of the second stage of labor. *Obstet Gynecol* 2009;113:1248–58.

12. American College of Obstetrics and Gynecology Committee of Practice Bulletins – Obstetrics. Practice Bulletin Number 49, December 2003: Dystocia and augmentation of labor. *Obstet Gynecol* 2003;102:1445–54.

4 Fetal surveillance in labour

In his 2007 annual report, the Chief Medical Officer of England expressed his concern about the static perinatal mortality rate in the UK over 7 years.[1] He highlighted the issue of intrapartum deaths in a chapter titled 'Intrapartum-Related Deaths: 500 Missed Opportunities'. These were cases where the fetus was alive on admission but died during labour. The incidence of intrapartum deaths has declined compared with 1995, when the fourth annual report of the Confidential Enquiry into Stillbirths and Deaths in Infancy reported intrapartum death in 1/1600 fetuses weighing more than 1500 g with no chromosomal or congenital malformation.[2] However, the factors that contributed to these deaths have not changed: inability to interpret the cardiotocograph (CTG) trace, failure to incorporate the 'clinical picture', delay in taking action and poor teamwork.

In addition to avoidable intrapartum fetal deaths, the incidence of hypoxic ischaemic encephalopathy (HIE) owing to birth asphyxia has not changed and remains about 2/1000, with 1/1000 being HIE grade I and the remainder being grades II and III. Grades II and III have a high correlation with asphyxia-related deaths and neurological injuries.[3] The mortality and morbidity related to intrapartum asphyxia affect the quality of life of parents and siblings and are an enormous drain on taxpayers, who indirectly contribute to the National Health Services Litigation Authority, which pays out billions of pounds in compensation for obstetric negligence in cases of intrapartum-related neurological injury. Currently, each case is awarded £3–6 million. Intrapartum hypoxia alone may contribute to 5–10% of cases of HIE, but intrapartum insult in cases with antenatal risk factors contributes to about 20–25% of cases of HIE.[4] The mechanism and type of brain injury at term attributable to asphyxia has been defined from animal models (see box overleaf).[5]

Acute total hypoxia that results in brainstem and thalamic injury gives rise to athetoid-type cerebral palsy. Partial prolonged hypoxia with acidosis is associated with cortical injury and results in spastic quadriparetic cerebral palsy. Magnetic resonance imaging studies of babies born at term who develop cerebral palsy have revealed that up to 28% of cases may be attributable to intrapartum-related asphyxia injuries.[6]

Recommendations for fetal monitoring in labour

Based on the evidence discussed above, the National Institute for Health and Clinical Excellence (NICE) has recommended continuous electronic fetal monitoring (EFM) for high-risk pregnancies and intermittent auscultation for low-risk women.[7]

INDICATIONS FOR THE USE OF CONTINUOUS EFM

Maternal
- Previous caesarean section
- Hypertension
- Post-term pregnancy (over 42 weeks)
- Prolonged rupture of membranes (over 24 hours)
- Induced labour
- Diabetes
- Antepartum haemorrhage
- Medical disorders, such as systemic lupus erythematosus

Fetal
- Fetal growth restriction
- Preterm gestation
- Oligohydramnios
- Abnormal umbilical artery Doppler velocimetry
- Multiple pregnancy
- Meconium-stained liquor
- Intrauterine infection

Intrapartum risk factors
- Oxytocin augmentation
- Epidural analgesia
- Vaginal bleeding in labour
- Maternal pyrexia
- Fresh meconium-stained liquor

Picker Institute Europe has established a patient-centred philosophy, which states that the patient should be involved in the management of their own health issues.[8] The same philosophy should be followed when offering fetal surveillance in labour: women should be offered the different methods of fetal surveillance available and the reason for recommending a preferred medical option explained.

Methods of intrapartum fetal monitoring

Monitoring should start with clinical evaluation of the pregnancy for risk factors: history, maternal vital parameters, symphyseal–fundal height and colour and quantity of amniotic fluid if the membranes are ruptured. Certain conditions predispose the fetus to develop acidosis more rapidly than a normally grown fetus at term with clear amniotic fluid. These conditions include preterm, post-term, fetal growth restriction, thick meconium with scant liquor, bleeding and infection. Iatrogenically, the fetus may be exposed to risk by injudicious use of oxytocin, difficult instrumental or breech delivery or macrosomia. Acute events such as placental abruption, scar rupture and cord prolapse should be clinically suspected and immediate action taken as the fetus is likely to be asphyxiated within a short period of time. Careful continuous surveillance should take place when administering epidural in the late first and second stage of labour, because a prolonged period of maternal thoracolumbar flexion with the fetal head deep in the pelvis can compromise uterine blood flow.

In the UK, the following options are available for fetal surveillance in labour:

- Intermittent auscultation of the fetal heart rate (FHR) using a fetal stethoscope or a Doptone device together with clinical palpation of contractions.

- EFM: continuous CTG by external transducers, for example ultrasound for the FHR and external pressure transducer to measure contractions. An internal scalp electrode for the FHR and an intrauterine pressure catheter to assess contractions are used where indicated.

- Fetal scalp blood sampling (FBS) for acid base as an adjunct to EFM.

- Fetal scalp lactate measurement.

- Fetal pulse oximetry.

- Fetal ECG-ST waveform analysis as an adjunct to CTG.

- Fetal stimulation tests.

INTERMITTENT AUSCULTATION

NICE recommends that the 'FHR should be auscultated every 15 minutes for a duration of 1 minute soon after a contraction during the first stage of labour and every 5 minutes or after every other contraction during the second stage of labour'.[7] The maternal pulse should be palpated and the fetal heart rate auscultated to differentiate between the maternal and fetal heart rates. In addition, the frequency and duration of contractions should be assessed by palpation and recorded on the partogram. The practice of intermittent auscultation should be taught and learned by medical students and midwifery students so that they are fully competent when they practise. In a low-risk labour, intermittent auscultation may need to be converted to EFM if there is meconium staining of the liquor, difficulty with auscultation or audible abnormality of the FHR, or if the labour needs augmentation with oxytocin. Some women at low risk may opt for EFM, which could be offered with the understanding that this may increase operative interventions and reduce the incidence of neonatal convulsions but not that of cerebral palsy.

CONTINUOUS EFM

Since the invention of autocorrelation technology (which accurately reflects baseline variability) in the 1980s, the Doppler ultrasound transducer has been increasingly used to acquire FHR signals. The transducer needs a light film of ultrasound jelly and is placed on the mother's abdomen over the region of the anterior shoulder of the fetus. If the external transducer does not give optimal signals (obese or restless mothers) or if fetal electrocardiogram (ECG) analysis is also to be evaluated, a fetal scalp electrode is applied to obtain fetal ECG signals to allow computation of the heart rate based on the RR interval of the ECG. Application of a scalp electrode is contraindicated if there is a bleeding disorder in the fetus or the mother has HIV or hepatitis B.

The frequency, duration and relative amplitude of uterine contractions are measured using a pressure gauge transducer placed on the abdomen between the uterine fundus and the umbilicus. With a uterine contraction the anteroposterior diameter of the uterus increases, which presses on the tocotransducer's diaphragm to record the uterine contraction. In rare circumstances, internal tocography using a strain-gauged catheter can be used, although there is little evidence to suggest that this is beneficial in induced or augmented labour.[9]

The fourth annual report on the Confidential Enquiry into Stillbirths and Death in Infancy highlighted the recurring problems related to incorrect interpretation of intrapartum FHR tracings.[2] Avoiding morbidity and mortality could be achieved only by having protocols for appropriate interpretation, adequate communication of the findings and timely clinical response for suspicious or pathological CTG. The clinical picture needs to be considered to allow appropriate action to be taken based on the CTG.

Since the introduction of EFM, there has been growing obstetric litigation based on the failure to perform prompt delivery in the presence of abnormal FHR patterns. To minimise errors in interpretation, NICE recommends that the settings on CTG machines should be standardised so that the paper speed is set to 1 cm/minute, sensitivity displays are set to 20 beats/minute (bpm)/cm and the FHR range displays of 50–210 bpm are used.[7]

The woman's name, hospital number, date of birth, pulse rate and temperature should always be checked before starting the recording, as should the date and time of the recording. The FHR should be auscultated by a fetal stethoscope or a Doppler device before starting EFM to avoid the maternal pulse being recorded by the fetal monitor. Ideally, both tocograph and cardiograph tracings should be clearly recorded in a continuous manner to provide a technically satisfactory trace. All intrapartum events (such as vaginal examination, fetal blood sample, epidural, mode of delivery) should be noted on the CTG. CTGs should be kept for a minimum of 25 years and therefore adequate provision should be available for the secure storage and easy retrieval of all CTGs.

Some hospitals in the UK incorporate central FHR monitoring into labour and delivery suites, which allows FHR patterns from different labouring women to be viewed simultaneously. This facilitates input from colleagues and senior personnel and may provide a higher level of vigilance, leading to a better perinatal outcome (similar to 'neighbourhood watch' schemes). This system also avoids medical personnel walking too often into rooms to review CTGs, which disturbs the privacy of the woman and her partner. However, the proven benefit of such a system remains inconclusive.

In women at high risk where continuous EFM is recommended in labour, the monitoring can be interrupted for short periods to permit the woman to use the shower or toilet if the CTG is normal. These interruptions are best avoided after any intervention that might alter the FHR, such as amniotomy, epidural insertion or top-up, or if the woman is receiving oxytocin infusion. Special caution must be exercised in women with previous caesarean scar, intrapartum bleeding or high fetal presenting part, where sudden sentinel events may occur that can compromise the fetus within a short period of time.

Admission CTG

Admission CTG has been proposed as a screening test to identify a fetus that is unable to tolerate labour, that is already hypoxic or that is likely to become hypoxic in labour.[10] Admission CTG is not recommended by NICE owing to insufficient evidence of maternal or fetal benefit. There is concern about the likelihood of prolonged FHR monitoring and immobilisation of women, which may result in more FBS and a possible increase in operative delivery rates. However, the admission test is still used in some units owing to the lack of midwifery staff available to provide optimal intermittent auscultation for 1 minute every 15 minutes in the first stage of labour.

Interpretation of CTG

FHR pattern recognition should be related to the uterine contractions. The four features of heart rate – baseline rate, baseline variability, accelerations and decelerations – should be classified. The whole trace should then be classified as normal, suspicious or pathological based on the individual features of the CTG. The characteristics needed to classify individual features as reassuring, non-reassuring and abnormal are given in Table 4.1.

The individual features of the CTG are first classified as reassuring, non-reassuring or abnormal (Table 4.2), followed by classification of the whole trace as normal, suspicious or pathological based on the four features of the CTG.

CLASSIFICATION OF CTG, TAKING INTO CONSIDERATION ALL FOUR FEATURES OF THE CTG ACCORDING TO THE NICE INTRAPARTUM CARE GUIDELINES[7]

- Normal: a CTG where all four features are classified as reassuring

- Suspicious: a CTG where one feature is classified as non-reassuring and the other features are classified as reassuring

- Pathological: a CTG where two or more features are classified as non-reassuring or one or more feature is classified as abnormal

---

A normal CTG is associated with a low probability of fetal compromise and has the following features: baseline rate 110–160 beats/minute; baseline variability of 5–25 beats/minute; accelerations of 15 beats/minute for 15 seconds x 2 in a 15-minute window (Figure 4.1). CTG in a term fetus with normal neurological behaviour will exhibit segments of

Table 4.1 Definitions and descriptions of individual features of fetal heart trace

Term	Definition
Baseline FHR	The mean FHR when stable, excluding accelerations and decelerations; determined over a period of 5–10 minutes and expressed in beats/minute
Normal baseline FHR	110–160 beats/minute
Moderate bradycardia	100–109 beats/minute
Moderate tachycardia	161–180 beats/minute
Abnormal bradycardia	Less than 100 beats/minute
Abnormal tachycardia	More than 180 beats/minute
Baseline variability	Minor fluctuations in baseline FHR occurring at three to five cycles/minute; measured by estimating the difference in beats/minute between highest peak and lowest trough of fluctuation in a 1-minute segment of the trace
Normal baseline variability	Greater than or equal to 5–25 beats/minute between contractions
Non-reassuring baseline variability	Less than 5 beats/minute for 40 minutes or more but less than 90 minutes
Abnormal baseline variability	Less than 5 beats/minute for 90 minutes or more
Accelerations	Transient increase in FHR of 15 beats/minute or more and lasting 15 seconds or more (Figure 4.1)
Decelerations	Transient episodes of slowing of FHR below the baseline level of more than 15 beats/minute and lasting 15 seconds or more
Early decelerations	Uniform, repetitive, periodic slowing of FHR with onset early in contraction and return to baseline at end of contraction (Figure 4.2)
Late decelerations	Uniform, repetitive, periodic slowing of FHR with onset of deceleration 20 seconds later than onset of contraction, or nadir of deceleration more than 20 seconds after peak of contraction, or end of deceleration 20 seconds after end of contraction; in the presence of a non-accelerative trace with baseline variability less than 5 beats/minute, the definition would include decelerations of less than 15 beats/minute (Figure 4.3)
Variable decelerations	Variable, intermittent, periodic slowing of FHR with rapid onset and recovery; time relationships with contraction cycles are variable and they may occur in isolation (Figure 4.4)
Prolonged decelerations	An abrupt decrease in FHR to under 80 beats/minute; suspicious if it lasts for less than 3 minutes and pathological if it lasts for more than 3 minutes
Sinusoidal pattern	A regular oscillation of the baseline resembling a sine wave with little baseline variability; this smooth, undulating pattern, lasting at least 10 minutes, has a relatively fixed period of three to five cycles/minute and an amplitude of 5–15 beats/minute above and below the baseline

Reproduced from guidelines collated by RCOG in association with NICE (2001).[10]

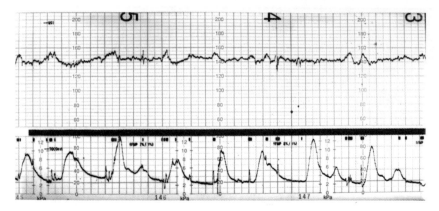

Figure 4.1 Reactive CTG with accelerations; an active and quiet epoch is also shown

no accelerations and reduced variability (quiet epochs) alternating with segments of accelerations and normal baseline variability (active epochs). The alternating of active and quiet epochs is called cycling. A fetus that had sustained neurological injury and recovered in the antenatal period may show sporadic accelerations, but cycling may be absent.

Maternal infection, with or without pyrexia, or a fetus with congenital or metabolic problems, hypoxia or cerebral haemorrhage may show a normal baseline rate but reduced baseline variability and no acceler-

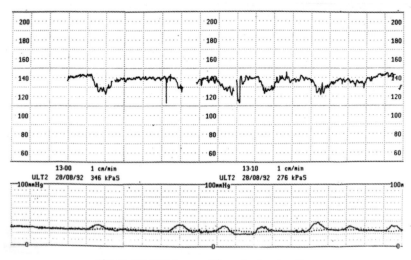

Figure 4.2 CTG trace with early decelerations

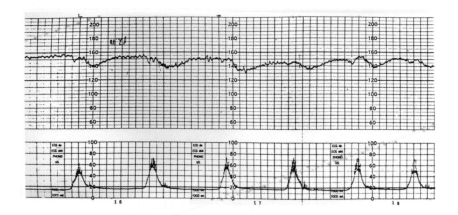

Figure 4.3 CTG trace with late decelerations

ations, which may result in a neonate with a low Apgar score and a poor prognosis. Compliance with guidelines and documentation with contemporaneous records is good practice. A CTG trace with minimal baseline variability, no accelerations and shallow decelerations is considered to depict a preterminal CTG trace and, possibly, pre-existing hypoxia (Figure 4.5) with a poor prognosis. A fetus with these characteristics is likely to present with one of the clinical features of infection, bleeding, thick meconium with scant fluid, severe pre-eclampsia, fetal growth restriction, post-term or absent fetal movements.

CTGs classified as suspicious or pathological need action to reverse the pattern to normal (such as change of maternal position, stopping oxytocin infusion and/or hydration), or just closer observation if the

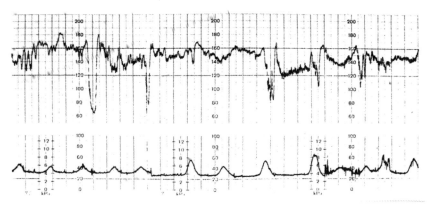

Figure 4.4 CTG trace with variable decelerations

Table 4.2 Classification of the individual FHR features (Intrapartum Care guidelines of the National Institute of Health and Clinical Excellence – NICE 2007)[7]

Feature	Baseline rate (beats/minute)	Variability	Decelerations	Accelerations
Reassuring (Figure 4.1)	110–160	≥ 5	None	Present
Non-reassuring	100–109 161–180	< 5 for > 40 minutes but < 90 minutes	Typical variable decelerations with > 50% of contractions occurring for > 90 minutes Single prolonged deceleration < 80 beats/minute for up to 3 minutes	The absence of accelerations with an otherwise normal CTG is of uncertain significance
Abnormal	< 100 > 180	< 5 for ≥ 90 minutes	Atypical variable or late or both types of decelerations occurring over 50% of contractions in a 30-minute period	
	Sinusoidal pattern for > 10 minutes		Single prolonged deceleration < 80 beats/minute for > 3 minutes	

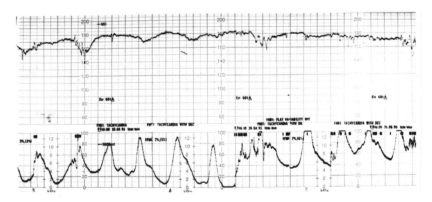

Figure 4.5 CTG trace suggestive of pre-existing hypoxia/preterminal trace

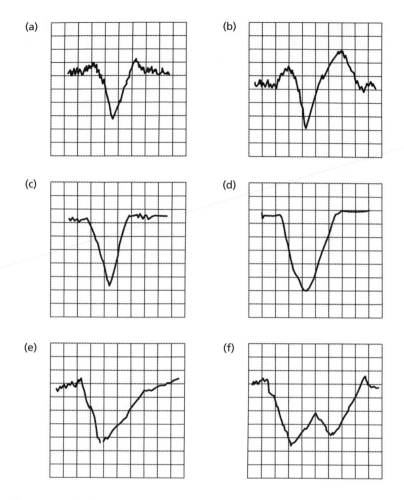

Figure 4.6 Variable decelerations: typical (a) and atypical (b–f): (a) typical variable with shouldering; (b) atypical with overshoot; (c) atypical with absence of shouldering; (d) atypical with duration over 60 seconds and depth over 60 seconds; (e) atypical with late recovery; (f) atypical with biphasic deceleration

situation is of no major concern (no clinical high-risk factors and only one abnormal feature). Further evaluation or the need to expedite delivery will be based on parity, cervical dilatation, rate of progress of labour, presence of high-risk factors and severity of the pathological trace. Acting solely based on the CTG increases operative delivery rates. The NICE guidelines recommend the use of FBS to measure the acid–base balance to increase specificity in the detection of fetuses that are likely to be compromised.

Some features in isolation do not signify compromise: baseline rate 00–109 beats/minute with normal baseline variability and accelertions but no decelerations; absence of accelerations; early decelerations ı the late first or second stage of labour; and simple variable decelertions. Atypical variable decelerations are abnormal and have features such as biphasic decelerations, for example variable followed by late recovery after the contraction, or deceleration that is over 60 beats in depth for longer than 60 seconds. Features of typical and atypical variable decelerations are shown in Figure 4.6.

CTG changes in labour may be a result of transient factors, such as maternal posture, amniotomy or hyperstimulation with oxytocics, or of inherent problems, including cord compression associated with oligohydramnios, placental insufficiency and fetal growth restriction. Alteration of position, hydration or stopping or reducing the oxytocics may help reverse the CTG changes. Sentinel events such as severe abruption, cord prolapse or scar rupture usually present with prolonged decelerations and need to be identified clinically and managed with immediate delivery.

Certain features in the CTG are more likely to be associated with fetal compromise. The chances of hypoxia and acidosis are greater with an increasing number of abnormal features: fetal tachycardia, reduced baseline variability less than 5 beats/minute for over 90 minutes, repeated complicated variable or late decelerations and prolonged decelerations lasting over 3 minutes. The extent of fetal compromise depends on the duration of the pathological pattern and the clinical status of the fetus. The longer the duration for which the FHR is below its normal baseline rate, the greater the chance of hypoxia. Persistent lack of baseline variability with a decelerative pattern denotes the possibility of acidosis.

A fetus with accelerations and normal baseline variability may develop variable decelerations with cord compression. With increasing hypoxia, the baseline rate increases (owing to a catecholamine surge), the decelerations become deeper and longer in duration and ultimately, after a rise in the baseline rate, the baseline variability decreases. If this pattern of gradually developing hypoxia continues, acidosis is likely. If no action is taken to improve the status of the fetus (for example altering the posture, stopping oxytocin/tocolysis and hydration), the FHR tends to gradually decrease, resulting in terminal bradycardia and fetal death.

In the presence of fetal tachycardia, one should exclude maternal pyrexia (with possible intrauterine infection), dehydration and the need for pain relief, especially if the CTG does not show any decelerations.

In clinical practice, preterminal CTGs are often overlooked. The CTG in such cases shows loss of variability and shallow decelerations in a non-reactive trace (Figure 4.5). The CTG that shows a total loss of variability with shallow decelerations is suggestive of a hypoxic fetus. Neurological damage may have already occurred and immediate delivery should be undertaken. Exposure to further uterine contractions may aggravate existing hypoxia, leading to more acidosis and its sequelae.

Immediate action should be considered with prolonged deceleration under 80 beats/minute for more than 3 minutes. This is a pathological CTG and suggests the possibility of acute hypoxia. In cases of severe abruption, cord prolapse, caesarean scar rupture and continuing prolonged deceleration, immediate delivery is warranted. In cases of prolonged deceleration in the absence of severe abruption, scar rupture and cord prolapse, the FHR tends to recover to its original baseline rate by 6 minutes in the vast majority of cases. While observing, one should prepare for delivery if the FHR does not show signs of recovery by 9 minutes.

A decision to deliver by 6 minutes may be appropriate in cases with a pathological CTG before prolonged deceleration and in cases with a particular vulnerability to hypoxia, such as thick meconium with scant fluid, fetal growth restriction, possible intrauterine infection, preterm, post-term and those with intrapartum bleeding. In other cases, the woman should be transferred to the operating theatre by 9 minutes if there are no signs of recovery. While awaiting recovery, oxytocin infusion should be stopped, the mother should be nursed in the left lateral position and one should consider hydration and acute short-acting tocolysis if there is evidence of uterine hyperstimulation. Ideally, caesarean section or instrumental vaginal delivery, when possible, should be commenced by 12 minutes with the aim of delivering the fetus by 15 minutes. Difficult instrumental deliveries should be avoided in such situations as the hypoxic fetal brain is more vulnerable to trauma.

Audits on decision-to-delivery interval or interval between onset of prolonged deceleration and delivery show that the usual delay is in transferring the woman to the theatre. Therefore, fire drills with practice runs for immediate deliveries and audit of cases of immediate delivery are recommended to help improve decision-to-delivery intervals.

FBS

EFM involves interpretation of FHR patterns. When the FHR shows two or more suspicious features or one or more pathological features, it is classified as pathological. The condition of the fetus with atypical variable decelerations, normal baseline rate and normal variability is pathological, but the condition of the fetus is likely to be better than that of a fetus with atypical variable decelerations, tachycardia and loss of baseline variability. The pathological features observed on the FHR trace, the clinical high-risk factors present, parity and the stage of labour may influence whether an immediate delivery or FBS is more suitable to manage the case. As EFM is a screening tool, the NICE guidelines recommend the use of FBS before caesarean delivery for a pathological trace to reduce unnecessary surgical intervention.

Known contraindications to FBS are maternal infections such as HIV, hepatitis B or C and herpes, fetal bleeding disorders such as haemophilia and preterm gestation (less than 34 weeks). FBS is contraindicated during prolonged deceleration as it will delay intervention if the FHR does not recover; also, the pH may be low owing to respiratory acidosis, which is corrected with the return of FHR to the baseline rate.

Using an amnioscope, a sample of blood (about 35 microlitres) is taken for blood gas analysis from the fetal scalp into a preheparinised capillary tube. FBS may be difficult to perform at cervical dilatations under 3 cm or when the head is high. A good-quality sample without contamination by amniotic fluid or trapping of air bubbles is needed for accurate measurement. Clinicians need to be trained on manikins to perform FBS as it is stressful for the mother if there is undue delay, which may also result in the blood clotting in the tube.

FBS is warranted based on the clinical situation and the CTG. Before FBS, corrective measures of positioning, stopping oxytocin infusion and hydration should be tried to restore the CTG to normal. The FBS results provide guidance for further management (Table 4.3). Immediate delivery is indicated if the pH is less than 7.20. FBS with pH over 7.25 is reassuring, but the trace should be observed. If CTG abnormalities persist, a repeat FBS is suggested after a suitable interval. If the CTG pattern gets worse, for example an increase in the duration and depth of deceleration, a rise in the baseline rate or a reduction in baseline variability, an earlier FBS is warranted. If the pH is in the pre-acidotic range (7.20–7.24), a repeat FBS is warranted within 30 minutes. If the pH is rapidly declining or is less than 7.20, delivery is recommended within 30 minutes. Confirmation of the condition of the fetus by umbilical arterial and venous blood pH at delivery in cases that undergo intrapartum FBS is good practice.

FETAL SCALP LACTATE MEASUREMENT

The fetal scalp blood sample can be subjected to lactate analysis, which is a direct measure of metabolic acidosis following hypoxia. The normal range needs to be established according to the equipment used.[11] Lactate measurements require 5 microlitres of blood compared with the 35 microlitres needed for measurement of pH and base excess. Using the

Table 4.3 Normal and abnormal values of pH and base excess

	pH	Base excess
Normal	>7.25	<–8 mmol/l
Suspicious	7.20–7.24	
Abnormal	<7.20	–12 mmol/l

Lactate Pro portable lactate meter (KDK Corporation, Kyoto, Japan), a fetal scalp level of 2.9–3.08 mmol/l should be considered suspicious and a level over 3.08 mmol as abnormal, warranting immediate intervention.[12] Lactate measurement is proving to be popular compared with pH measurement because the failure rate of obtaining a sample for analysis is significantly less than for pH and base excess.[13] Umbilical arterial lactate levels correlate well with pH and base excess, and a two-year follow-up of neonates and a Cochrane review recommend the use of lactate measurement in clinical practice.[14]

FETAL PULSE OXIMETRY

Continuous measurement of fetal oxygen saturation by pulse oximetry from the fetus has been made possible with the use of special sensors. Measurements are taken using different wavelengths and the knowledge of differential absorption of the light by deoxygenated and oxygenated haemoglobin. A comparison of the measurements with the standard curves of the oximeter helps to determine fetal oxygen saturation. The sensor is inserted via the vagina and placed in direct contact with the fetal cheek/scalp.

Sensors in a diaphragm at the base of the standard scalp electrode have been developed and are being successfully used. The sensor is connected to a conventional heart rate monitor and the oxygen saturation is continuously plotted against the 0–100 scale of the tocodynamometer tracing of the conventional CTG paper. The normal fetal oxygen saturation fluctuates between 30% and 80% and the fetus does not develop acidosis unless the oxygen saturation is less than 30% over a 10-minute period.[15] Normal oxygen saturation measurements indicate fetal health. However, the difficulty in obtaining satisfactory readings over 90% of the time in 90% of labours, and the failure to show improvement in neonatal outcome or reduction in operative vaginal delivery rates, have made this a method to be used in research settings only. Based on the 2007 Cochrane review, it is not recommended for clinical use.[16]

FETAL ECG-ST WAVEFORM ANALYSIS

ST changes observed with myocardial strain during exercise are used in human adults to diagnose the possibility of myocardial ischaemia. Early animal studies with fetal lambs have shown ST changes with hypoxia. Subsequent studies have shown that human fetuses exhibit similar changes and that ECG waveform analysis can be used as an adjunct to CTG in detecting fetal hypoxia.[17]

The catecholamine stress of hypoxia leads to myocardial glycogen-olysis. The liberated glucose enters the myocardial cells with the potassium ions, causing ST changes. These changes are measured as T/QRS ratios (Figure 4.7) and could manifest as an episodic rise or a steady continuing rise in the T/QRS ratio. When there is a less refractory period for the myocardium to repolarise, the ST segment is distorted and could be above (grade I biphasic ST), cutting (grade II biphasic) or below (grade III biphasic) the isoelectric line (Figure 4.8).

Electronic technology has advanced, leading to automated ST analysis, which is increasingly being used as an adjunct to CTG when the CTG shows a suspicious trace and/or in high-risk pregnancies. The fetal ECG is obtained using a single spiral scalp electrode and a reference maternal skin electrode. Thirty raw ECG signals are averaged into a single ECG for analysis. The T/QRS is plotted as a cross on the CTG paper on a scale of 0.0–0.50 just below the tocodynamometer channel and is also displayed on the screen. The baseline T/QRS ratio is calculated in the first 20 minutes; any subsequent rise is calculated by the computer and displayed as an ST event (Figure 4.9). Continuous recording is advised as significant ST events could be missed if the electrode or machine is

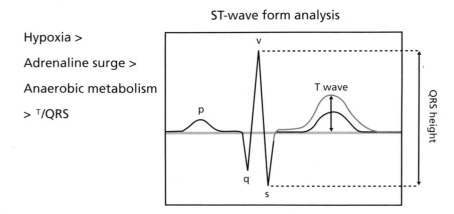

Figure 4.7 ECG waveform changes with hypoxia and adrenaline surge

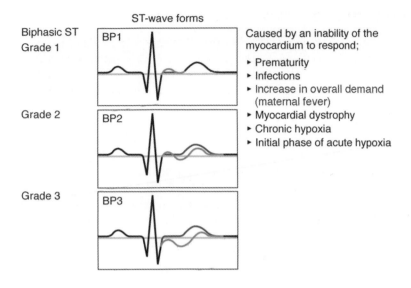

ST-wave forms

Biphasic ST Grade 1	BP1	Caused by an inability of the myocardium to respond;
		▸ Prematurity
		▸ Infections
		▸ Increase in overall demand (maternal fever)
Grade 2	BP2	▸ Myocardial dystrophy
		▸ Chronic hypoxia
		▸ Initial phase of acute hypoxia
Grade 3	BP3	

Figure 4.8 Biphasic ST waveforms

disconnected for more than 4 minutes. The type and magnitude of ECG change (episodic rise, continuous baseline rise or biphasic change: Table 4.4), the CTG changes observed and the clinical picture determine the type of clinical intervention.

Table 4.4 Guidelines for the use of CTG and STAN based on the type and magnitude of ECG change

ST events	Normal CTG	Intermediary/ suspicious CTG	Abnormal CTG
Episodic T/QRS rise	Expectant management	> 0.15	> 0.10
Baseline T/QRS rise	Continued observation	> 0.10	> 0.05
Biphasic ST		Three biphasic log messages	Two biphasic log messages

These guidelines may indicate situations where obstetric interventions may be required.
- Pre-terminal CTG (prolonged deceleration or CTG with no variability and decelerations): immediate delivery required.
- Intervention may include delivery or maternofetal resuscitation by alleviating contributing problems such as overstimulation or maternal hypotension or hypoxia.
- The time span between the biphasic messages should be related to the CTG pattern and the clinical situation.

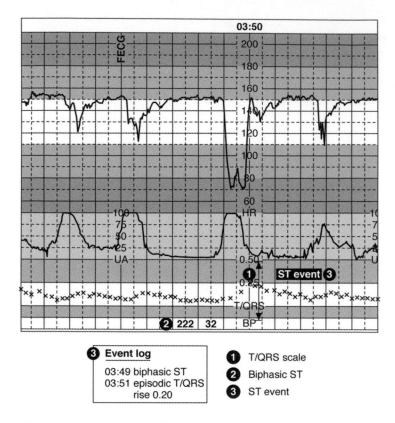

Figure 4.9 CTG and ST waveform analysis with ST event logs shown on screen

Meta-analysis of studies on fetal ECG-ST waveform analysis suggests that, when used as an adjunct to CTG, this technique can reduce the incidence of FBS, metabolic acidosis and neonatal convulsions.[18] The literature has highlighted that occasionally the fetus can become hypoxic and acidotic without changes in the ST waveform although the CTG may become preterminal.[19] In light of these reports, a European expert group revised the guidelines for the use of fetal ECG waveform analysis in labour.[20] The CTG interpretation is based on the International Federation of Gynecology and Obstetrics classification,[21] which is slightly different from the NICE classification of CTG.[7]

ST waveform analysis is not used for fetuses at less than 36 weeks of gestation owing to the number of biphasic events with little significance. Biphasic events have also been observed with maternal infection/ pyrexia and congenital heart defects. At times, ST changes are seen with a normal reactive CTG when no action is warranted. If the CTG is preterminal (no baseline variability and shallow late decelerations: Figure 4.5) or there is prolonged deceleration less than 80 beats/minute for more than 3 minutes, prompt delivery should be undertaken without awaiting ST changes. If the CTG is pathological for more than 60 minutes with no ST changes, a review by a senior colleague is mandated. In the second stage of labour, if the CTG is pathological for more than 60 minutes, assisted vaginal delivery is recommended despite no ST changes, as sudden deterioration of the CTG may occur with little time available to intervene.

FETAL STIMULATION TESTS

Acceleration at the time of scalp blood sampling is the basis of stimulation tests; spontaneous and provoked accelerations are associated with a non-acidotic fetus.[22] The fetus that does not accelerate from the stimulus has a 50% chance of being acidotic.[23]

A fetal acoustic stimulation test is recommended by the American College of Obstetricians and Gynecologists as an adjunctive test in fetal surveillance.[24] If FBS is not feasible, the decision should be made to deliver the fetus or observe based on the severity of the pathological CTG and the clinical background factors.

Conclusion

Injury to the fetus from birth asphyxia is an event that can be prevented in many cases by careful management of labour with good interpretation of the CTG and appropriate action in relation to the clinical context. Adjuncts of pH, lactate and ECG waveform analysis are of value but care needs to be exercised in the proper use of these techniques. The RCOG, the RCM and e-Learning for Healthcare are developing an electronic tool to provide education and training in CTG interpretation and appropriate action. Current research, including the INFANT trial using computer interpretation of CTG and the Euro CisPorto trial of computer interpretation of CTG with ECG waveform analysis, may provide better technology in the future to reduce the incidence of birth asphyxia and operative delivery for 'fetal distress'.

CLINICIAN'S GUIDE TO INTERPRETATION OF CTG[25]

- Accelerations and normal baseline variability are hallmarks of fetal health.
- Accelerations with reduced baseline variability are probably of little concern.
- Periods of decreased variability may represent fetal sleep.
- Hypoxic fetuses may have a normal baseline rate between 110 beats/minute and 160 beats/minute with no accelerations and baseline variability less than 5 beats/minute for over 40 minutes.
- With baseline variability under 5 beats/minute, even shallow decelerations less than 15 beats/minute are ominous with a non-reactive CTG.
- Placental abruption, cord prolapse and scar rupture can give rise to acute hypoxia and should be identified and dealt with clinically.
- Hypoxia and acidosis may develop faster with an abnormal trace in women with scant thick meconium, fetal growth restriction, intrauterine infection with pyrexia and those who are preterm or post-term.
- In preterm fetuses (especially less than 34 weeks of gestation), hypoxia and acidosis can predispose to hyaline membrane disease and respiratory distress syndrome and may contribute to intraventricular haemorrhage and its sequelae, warranting early action in the presence of a pathological trace.
- Injudicious use of oxytocin, epidural anaesthesia and difficult deliveries can worsen hypoxia.
- During labour, if decelerations are absent, asphyxia is unlikely but cannot be excluded.
- Abnormal patterns may represent not only hypoxia but also effects of drugs, fetal anomaly, infection or cerebral haemorrhage.

References

1. Intrapartum-Related Deaths: 500 Missed Opportunities. In: Department of Health. *On the state of public health: Annual report of the Chief Medical Officer 2006*. London: Department of Health; 2007 [www.dh.gov.uk/en/ Publicationsandstatistics/Publications/AnnualReports/DH_076817].
2. Maternal and Child Health Research Consortium. *Confidential Enquiry into Stillbirths and Deaths in Infancy: 4th Annual Report, 1 January–31 December 1995*. London: Maternal and Child Health Research Consortium, 1997.
3. Kjellmer I, Beijer E, Carlsson G, Hrbek A, Viggedal G. Follow-up into young adulthood after cardiopulmonary resuscitation in term and near-term newborn infants. I. Educational achievements and social adjustment. *Acta Paediatr* 2002;91:1212–17.

4. Badawi N, Kurinczuk JJ, Keogh JM, Alessandrini LM, O'Sullivan F, Burton PR, et al. Intrapartum risk factors for newborn encephalopathy: the Western Australian case–control study. *BMJ* 1998;317:1554–8.

5. Myers RE. Brain damage due to asphyxia: mechanism of causation. *J Perinat Med* 1981;9 Suppl 1:78–86.

6. Hagberg B, Hagberg G, Beckung E, Uvebrant P. Changing panorama of cerebral palsy in Sweden. VIII. Prevalence and origin in the birth year period 1991–94. *Acta Paediatr* 2001;90:271–7.

7. National Institute for Health and Clinical Excellence. *Intrapartum care. Care of healthy women and their babies during childbirth*. NICE clinical guideline 55, London: NICE; 2007 [http://guidance.nice.org.uk/CG55].

8. Picker Institute Europe. *"No decisions about me, without me." Annual Review 2009/10*. Oxford: Picker Institute Europe; 2010 [http://www.pickereurope. org/item/document/282].

9. Badder JJ, Verhoeven CJ, Janssen PF, van Lith JM, van Oudgaarden ED, Bloemenkamp KW, et al. Outcomes after internal versus external tocodynamometry for monitoring labor. *N Engl J Med* 2010;362:306–13.

10. Ingemarsson I, Arulkumaran S, Ingemarsson E, Tambyraja RL, Ratnam SS, Admission test: a screening test for fetal distress in labor. *Obstet Gynecol* 1986;68:800–6.

11. Nordström L, Chua S, Roy A, Arulkumaran S. Quality assessment of two lactate strip methods for obstetric use. *J Perinat Med* 1998;26:83–8.

12. Nordström L, Arulkumaran S. Intrapartum fetal hypoxia and biochemical markers: a review. *Obstet Gynecol Surv* 1998;53:645–57.

13. Westgren M, Kruger K, Ek S, Grunevald C, Kublickas M, Naka K, et al. Lactate compared with pH analysis at fetal scalp blood sampling: a prospective randomised study. *Br J Obstet Gynaecol* 1998;105:29–33.

14. East CE, Leader LR, Sheehan P, Henshall NE, Colditz PB. Intrapartum fetal scalp lactate sampling for fetal assessment in the presence of a non-reassuring fetal heart rate trace. *Cochrane Database Syst Rev* 2010;(3):CD006174.

15. Chua S, Yeong SM, Razvi K, Arulkumaran S. Fetal oxygen saturation during labour. *Br J Obstet Gynaecol* 1997;104:1080–3.

16. East CE, Chan FY, Colditz PB, Begg LM. Fetal pulse oximetry for fetal assessment in labour. *Cochrane Database Syst Rev* 2007;(2):CD004075.

17. Arulkumaran S, Lilja H, Lindecrantz K, Ratnam SS, Thavarasah A, Rosén KG. Fetal ECG waveform analysis should improve fetal surveillance in labour. *J Perinat Med* 1990;18:13–22.

18. Neilson JP. Fetal electrocardiogram (ECG) for fetal monitoring during labour. *Cochrane Database Syst Rev* 2006;(3):CD000116.

19. Doria V, Papageorghiou AT, Gustaffson A, Ugwumadu A, Farrer K, Arulkumaran S. Review of the first 1502 cases of ECG-ST waveform analysis during labour in a teaching hospital. *BJOG* 2007;114:1202–7.

20. Amer-Wahlin I, Arulkumaran S, Hagberg H, Marsál K, Visser GH. Fetal electrocardiogram: ST waveform analysis in intrapartum surveillance. *BJOG* 2007;114:1191–3.

21. Intrapartum surveillance: recommendations on current practice and overview of new developments. FIGO Study Group on the Assessment of New Technology. International Federation of Gynecology and Obstetrics. *Int J Gynaecol Obstet* 1995;49:213–21.
22. Clark SL, Gimovsky ML, Miller FC. The scalp stimulation test: a clinical alternative to fetal scalp blood sampling. *Am J Obstet Gynecol* 1984;148:274–7.
23. Arulkumaran S, Ingemarsson I, Ratnam SS. Fetal heart rate response to scalp stimulation as a test of fetal well-being in labour. *Asia Oceania J Obstet Gynaecol* 1987;13:131–5.
24. American College of Obstetricians and Gynecologists. ACOG Practice Bulletin No. 106: Intrapartum fetal heart rate monitoring: nomenclature, interpretation, and general management principles. American College of Obstetricians and Gynecologists. *Obstet Gynecol* 2009;114:192–202.
25. Arulkumaran S, Ingemarsson I, Montan S, Gibb D, Paul, RH, Schiffrin B, Spencer JA, Steer PJ, van Geijn HP. *Clinician's Guide: Traces of you – Fetal Trace Interpretation*. Germany: Philips; 2002 [www.healthcare.philips.com/main/products/mother_and_child_care/pre_natal_care/id_care/homePage.wpd].

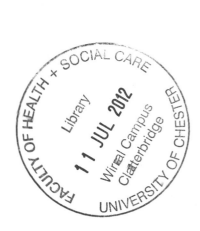

5 Third stage of labour

The third stage of labour lasts from the birth of the infant until delivery of the placenta. It usually lasts for 5–10 minutes and rarely more than 30 minutes. Although it is the shortest of the three stages of labour, it carries the greatest potential risk for the mother.

Physiology

After delivery of the infant, the uterus continues to contract rhythmically. The muscle fibres of the uterus, which have stretched considerably to accommodate the fetus, are shortened dramatically by these contractions and sustained by retraction. Retraction is the property unique to the uterus, by which muscle fibre length is permanently shortened after the active, energy-consuming contraction has passed.

PLACENTAL SEPARATION

Contraction and retraction of the uterine muscle cause a progressive reduction in the size of the placental implantation site. Thus, the relatively inelastic placenta buckles and is sheared from the uterine wall. An additional but much less significant role involves compression of the decidual veins by the uterine contraction, while the spiral arteries continue to pump blood into the intervillous space. This extravasation of blood helps dissect through the decidua spongiosa layer. Once the placenta has physically separated from the uterine wall, the myometrial contractions assist the passage of the placenta from the uterine cavity, through the cervix and into the upper vagina.

HAEMOSTASIS

Separation of the placenta leaves a very vascular placental bed with torn blood vessels. However, the uterine muscle fibres are arranged in a crisscross fashion and the vessels pass through this latticework. As a result, when the uterine muscle contracts, the vessels are effectively compressed by these 'physiological sutures' or 'living ligatures'. This anatomical and physiological mechanism is one of the haemostatic marvels of the human body (Figure 5.1).

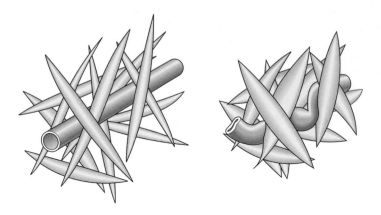

Figure 5.1 Haemostatic mechanism after placental delivery: 'living ligatures' or 'physiological sutures'

SIGNS OF PLACENTAL SEPARATION

There are three clinical signs of placental separation:

- The uterine fundus rises and changes from a broad discoid shape to a more narrow globular form as a result of the placenta separating and leaving the upper uterine segment.
- As the edge of the placenta separates from the uterine wall, bleeding will occur, usually as a fairly brisk gush of blood. This is not a completely reliable sign as bleeding may start when only part of the placenta has separated or, conversely, may not be seen at all when the entire placenta has separated but the blood is contained behind the membranes.
- Cord lengthening of 8–15 cm is the most reliable sign of placental separation.

Management

After delivery of the infant, the cord is clamped and divided and appropriate cord blood samples are collected. Unless there is a compelling need for neonatal resuscitation, cord clamping should be delayed for 1–2 minutes to reduce anaemia in the newborn.[1]

The woman is then closely observed for signs of placental separation. While waiting for these signs, the attendant places the cord clamp at the level of the introitus so that cord lengthening can be appreciated. One hand should cradle and guard the fundus to appreciate the uterine signs of placental separation or, alternatively, to aid early detection of an atonic uterus filling with blood. The uterine hand should not manipulate the fundus as interference may increase blood loss or stimulate a constriction ring, causing retained placenta. When the clinical signs of separation occur, the attendant delivers the placenta by controlled cord traction. For this manoeuvre, one hand is placed on the lower part of the uterus just above the symphysis and presses gently upwards and backwards as steady traction with the other hand on the clamp delivers the placenta (Figure 5.2). The placenta is then carefully examined to ensure it is complete.

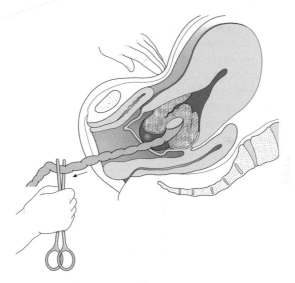

Figure 5.2 Delivery of the placenta by controlled cord traction

There are two approaches to the routine management of the third stage of labour: expectant or physiological management and active management.

EXPECTANT OR PHYSIOLOGICAL MANAGEMENT

In essence, expectant or physiological management entails waiting for the normal physiological changes that bring about placental separation and haemostasis. This approach is favoured by women and their attendants who prefer limited intervention in the management of labour. Some will encourage immediate suckling after birth to reduce blood loss and postpartum haemorrhage.[2] Unfortunately, compared with active management, this physiologically attractive approach is associated with three times the risk of atonic postpartum haemorrhage of over 1000 ml (2.6% compared with 0.9%).[3] Active management reduces the duration of the third stage by almost 50%, from about 16 minutes with the expectant approach to approximately 9 minutes with active management.[3]

ACTIVE MANAGEMENT

Active management involves giving an oxytocic drug at or just after delivery of the infant to induce an early and consistent uterine contraction, thereby producing placental separation and haemostasis without delay. Atonic postpartum haemorrhage, the most common complication of the third stage of labour, is dealt with in chapter 19. Routine active management of the third stage of labour is aimed at preventing the occurrence of atonic postpartum haemorrhage. Randomised controlled trials have consistently shown that blood loss, postpartum haemorrhage and the need for blood transfusion are all reduced by 40–60% when active is compared with expectant management.[4–6] Active management using oxytocin does not increase the risk of retained placenta, nor does it increase nausea and vomiting. Ergometrine does increase the incidence of nausea and vomiting and in some, but not all, studies predisposed women to retained placenta.[7,8] Thus, the evidence in favour of active management is now conclusive and this method should be accepted as the standard of care, unless the woman specifically wishes to have no intervention. Furthermore, a comparison between administration of the oxytocic before and after delivery of the placenta shows a clear reduction in postpartum haemorrhage when the oxytocic is given before placental delivery.[9]

Active management of the third stage of labour has been endorsed as the standard of care by the World Health Organization, the International Federation of Gynecology and Obstetrics, the International Confederation of Midwives and most national obstetric societies.[10–13] The elements of active management endorsed by these groups include:

- ten units of oxytocin by intramuscular injection within 1 minute of delivery
- clamp and divide the cord 1–3 minutes after delivery
- deliver the placenta by controlled cord traction after signs of placental separation
- massage the uterus to ensure it remains contracted.

In the first few hours postpartum, the woman is also vulnerable to uterine atony and haemorrhage. Close observation, particularly for the first 2–3 hours after delivery, is therefore essential. During this time the uterus should be regularly massaged to ensure that it is well contracted. As a full bladder can interfere with uterine retraction, the bladder should be kept empty. If an intravenous drip is already in place, the addition of 20 units of oxytocin to 500 ml of crystalloid will assist in maintaining uterine contractions. If ergometrine or Syntometrine® (Alliance Pharmaceuticals Ltd, Chippenham, UK) has been used, the more prolonged effect of these drugs usually accomplishes the maintenance of uterine contractions without further doses. No part of active management of labour need interfere with the new parents' involvement with and attachment to their new baby.

Oxytocic drugs

The characteristics of the available oxytocic drugs are outlined below and summarised in Table 5.1.

OXYTOCIN

Oxytocin is the cheapest and safest oxytocic drug. It produces rapid, rhythmic uterine contractions lasting for 15–30 minutes. The dose is five units intravenously, ten units intramuscularly or via intravenous infusion, such as 20 units in 500 ml crystalloid. Oxytocin has transient relaxant effects on vascular smooth muscle. It may produce a mild but clinically insignificant reduction in blood pressure as a result of reduced total peripheral resistance.[14,15] For this reason, the intravenous dose may be given over 2–3 minutes rather than as a rapid bolus. Because of its safety and lack of contraindications, oxytocin is the oxytocic drug of first choice.

ERGOMETRINE

Having been in use for 75 years, ergometrine has pride of place in the history of prevention and management of postpartum haemorrhage.[16] Ergometrine induces prolonged uterine contractions for 60–120 minutes. It produces peripheral vasoconstriction which, in the normal woman, is usually not clinically significant. However, in women with pre-eclampsia or chronic hypertension, this effect can be pronounced and precipitate a hypertensive crisis or eclamptic fit. Ergometrine is therefore contraindicated in all patients with hypertensive disease. Ergometrine-induced vasoconstriction is responsive to intravenous chlorpromazine or glyceryl

Table 5.1 Oxytocic drugs

Drug	Dose and route	Duration of action	Adverse effects	Contraindications
Oxytocin	5 units IV 10 units IM 20 units in 500 ml infusion	15–30 minutes	Insignificant hypotension and flushing, water intoxication in high doses (more than 200 units)	None
Ergometrine	0.2–0.25 mg IM or IV	1–2 hours	Nausea, vomiting, hypertension, vasospasm	Pre-eclampsia/ hypertension, cardiovascular disease
Syntometrine®* (5 units oxytocin, 0.5 mg ergometrine)	1 ampoule IM	1–2 hours	Nausea, vomiting, hypertension, vasospasm	Pre-eclampsia/ hypertension, cardiovascular disease
15-methyl prostaglandin F2α (Hemabate®**)	0.25 mg IM or IMM 0.25 mg in 500 ml infusion	4–6 hours	Vomiting, diarrhoea, flushing, shivering, pyrexia, vasospasm, bronchospasm	Cardiovascular disease, asthma
Carbetocin	100 micrograms IM or IV	2 hours	Flushing	None
Misoprostol	400–600 micrograms sublingual or oral	1–2 hours	Nausea, diarrhoea, shivering, pyrexia	None

* Alliance Pharmaceuticals Ltd, Chippenham, UK; **Pharmacia, Pfizer Ltd, New York, USA; IM = intramuscular; IMM = intramyometrial; IV = intravenous

trinitrate. On very rare occasions ergometrine can induce coronary artery spasm, and isolated cases of myocardial infarction have been attributed to its use. In the context of the millions of women who have received ergometrine, such cases are incredibly rare. Coronary artery spasm induced by ergometrine should respond to intravenous glyceryl trinitrate. Nausea and vomiting is also a common adverse effect of ergometrine, occurring in up to 20–25% of women. The dose of ergometrine is 0.2–0.25 mg, preferably by intramuscular injection, but if the need is urgent it can be given as a slow intravenous bolus.

SYNTOMETRINE

Syntometrine is a combination of five units of oxytocin and 0.5 mg of ergometrine and thus combines the rapid onset of oxytocin with the more prolonged effect of ergometrine. Syntometrine carries the same complications and contraindications as ergometrine, although the mild vasodilatation effect of oxytocin may to some extent ameliorate the vasopressor effect of ergometrine.

15-METHYL PROSTAGLANDIN F2α

The 15-methyl analogue of prostaglandin F2α (carboprost, Hemabate®; Pharmacia, Pfizer Ltd, New York, USA) has a much stronger uterotonic effect than its parent compound, resulting in good oxytocic action with less of the undesirable smooth-muscle stimulatory effects (vasoconstriction, bronchoconstriction, nausea and vomiting). Flushing, shivering and pyrexia (37.5–38.5°C) are not uncommon but relatively mild adverse effects. The dose is 0.25 mg intramuscularly or intramyometrially. Most authors agree that an intravenous bolus should be avoided because of the possibility of more profound smooth-muscle stimulation adverse effects, although 15-methyl prostaglandin F2α has been used many times by that route without ill effect. For rapid onset the intramyometrial route is preferred. This is achieved by diluting the 1 ml ampoule containing 0.25 mg of 15-methyl prostaglandin F2α in 5 ml normal saline and injecting this transabdominally using a 20-gauge spinal needle into two sites in the uterine fundus. The duration of action is up to 6 hours. This drug has proved very valuable as a second-line agent in cases of uterine atony unresponsive to oxytocin and ergometrine.[17,18] 15-methyl prostaglandin F2α can also be given as a dilute solution of 0.25 mg in 500 ml saline and administered as an infusion.[19]

CARBETOCIN

Carbetocin is a synthetic analogue of oxytocin with a duration of action of up to 2 hours. The dose is 100 micrograms, which can be given either intramuscularly or as a slow bolus by intravenous injection. Carbetocin is more expensive than oxytocin but can be used as an alternative to a continuous oxytocin infusion.[20] The adverse effects of carbetocin (flushing and mild hypotension) are similar to those of oxytocin.

MISOPROSTOL

An analogue of prostaglandin E1, misoprostol has many qualities that make it attractive for low-resource settings. It is cheap, stable at extremes of temperature and has a long shelf life. The duration of action is about 2 hours.

Misoprostol is the only uterotonic drug that can be given by the non-parenteral route: it can be given orally, sublingually, vaginally or rectally, depending on the clinical situation. Misoprostol is more effective than placebo for the prevention of postpartum haemorrhage but slightly less effective than the injectable oxytocic drugs.[21,22] For the prevention of postpartum haemorrhage, the dose is 400–600 micrograms either sublingually or orally. Misoprostol is also valuable as a second-line uterotonic when oxytocin fails. For the treatment of haemorrhage, the usual dose is 800 micrograms sublingually or 1000 micrograms rectally.

Retained placenta

There is evidence from ultrasound studies that, in addition to a generalised uterine contraction, there is a specific retroplacental myometrial contraction that is essential for complete placental separation. Retained placenta is more common in preterm and induced labours and the retroplacental myometrial contraction is more likely to be absent in these cases.[23,24] There is no international consensus on the definition of retained placenta. With expectant management of the third stage of labour, the placenta is usually delivered within 10–20 minutes; with active management, this time is halved. The incidence of retained placenta 30 minutes after delivery of the infant is about 2–4%, and half this value at 60 minutes following delivery. In general, the longer the duration of the third stage beyond 30 minutes, the greater the likelihood of haemorrhage and the less likely spontaneous delivery of the placenta. In most cases the treatment is manual removal of the placenta under anaesthesia. Thus, in the absence of active bleeding, the decision when to proceed to manual removal depends to a large extent on the availability of safe anaesthesia. If the patient has regional anaesthesia in place for delivery, there is little to be gained by waiting longer than 15–20 minutes before proceeding to manual removal. If, however, anaesthesia has to be induced, most will wait for 30 minutes and then marshal the resources to provide anaesthesia. This usually takes 20–30 minutes so that manual removal is usually performed about 60 minutes after delivery of the infant. By waiting between 30 and 60 minutes, the placenta will deliver spontaneously in 50% of these cases. Obviously, this slower approach to manual removal is valid only if there is no active bleeding. If haemorrhage supervenes, immediate steps to remove the placenta must be taken.

CAUSES OF RETAINED PLACENTA

The placenta that has separated from the uterine wall may be retained owing to uterine atony or the presence of a uterine constriction ring.

Retained adherent placenta can be a result of ordinary adherence with failure of separation through the decidua spongiosa layer, or of pathological adherence owing to a deficient decidual reaction allowing invasion of the myometrium by the trophoblast. The latter is more likely in a uterine site previously affected by surgery, trauma or infection. It is rare for the entire placental surface to be pathologically adherent, but areas of partial accreta will be encountered.

The placenta that is praevia is more likely to be pathologically adherent because of the poor decidual response of the lower uterine segment. This is discussed in chapter 18, page 202.

MANAGEMENT OF RETAINED PLACENTA

If the retained placenta is associated with uterine atony or a constriction ring, haemorrhage is more likely. If haemorrhage occurs, the bleeding is treated with intravenous oxytocin and steps are taken to deliver the placenta. In selected cases when anaesthesia is not in place and the placenta is thought to be separated but retained because of a constriction ring, glyceryl trinitrate can be used to aid spontaneous delivery of the placenta without the need for anaesthesia and manual removal.[25] Obviously, in such cases one has to have everything set up so that if the nitroglycerin does not work, anaesthesia can be induced to allow manual removal without delay.

Ultimately, if these measures fail or are not suitable, the management of retained placenta is manual removal (Figure 5.3). Timing and anaesthetic considerations have already been discussed.

TECHNIQUE FOR MANUAL REMOVAL OF THE PLACENTA

After induction of suitable anaesthesia, place one well-lubricated hand in the vagina and follow the cord up through the cervix. With the other hand, firmly cradle and push down on the uterine fundus.

The fingers and thumb of the uterine hand should be kept extended and used as one unit to find the lower margin of the placenta and, with side-to-side movements, find and separate through the plane of cleavage. Once the placenta has been completely separated, it should be grasped and slowly removed through the cervix. It is important not to do this too rapidly as it is possible to invert the uterus if part of the placenta remains adherent. Once the placenta has been removed, the uterus is re-explored to make sure that there are no remaining placental fragments and that the uterine wall is intact. In cases where there are small areas of pathological adherence, the placenta should be removed piecemeal from those sites. The cervix and vagina should be checked, and any lacerations sutured.

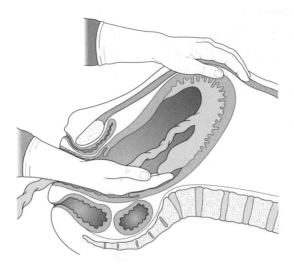

Figure 5.3 Manual removal of the placenta

Run an intravenous infusion of oxytocin in crystalloid to maintain uterine contraction and retraction.

A broad-spectrum antibiotic may be given for 24 hours to prevent infection.

With regional anaesthesia there may not be sufficient uterine relaxation to allow access of the hand into the uterus. In such cases, intravenous glyceryl trinitrate may be used (see chapter 23 for details of its administration).

INTRAUMBILICAL INJECTION OF OXYTOCIN

In some cases of retained placenta, injection into the umbilical cord vein of 10–30 units of oxytocin mixed in 20–30 ml normal saline has been used to aid delivery of the placenta. It was postulated that the delivery of oxytocin to the placental bed would induce the retroplacental myometrial contraction necessary to separate the placenta.[22] Unfortunately, in a randomised controlled trial, this simple and safe procedure was not found to be effective using oxytocin.[26] Studies using larger volumes and different oxytocics are under way.[27]

The remaining complications of the third stage of labour are covered in chapter 19.

References

1. Hutton EK, Hassan ES. Late vs early clamping of the umbilical cord in full-term neonates: systematic review and meta-analysis of controlled trials. *JAMA* 2007;297:1241–52.
2. Chua S, Arulkumaran S, Lim I, Selamat N, Ratnam SS. Influence of breastfeeding and nipple stimulation on postpartum uterine activity. *Br J Obstet Gynaecol* 1994;101:804–5.
3. Prendiville WJ, Elbourne D, McDonald S. Active versus expectant management in the third stage of labour. *Cochrane Database Syst Rev* 2000;(3):CD000007.
4. Prendiville W, Elbourne D, Chalmers I. The effects of routine oxytocic administration in the management of the third stage of labour: an overview of the evidence from controlled trials. *Br J Obstet Gynaecol* 1988;95:3–16.
5. Rogers J, Wood J, McCandlish R, Ayres S, Truesdale A, Elbourne D. Active versus expectant management of the third stage of labour: the Hinchingbrooke randomised controlled trial. *Lancet* 1998;351:693–9.
6. Rajan PV, Wing DA. Postpartum hemorrhage: evidence-based medical interventions for prevention and treatment. *Clin Obstet Gynecol* 2010;53:165–81.
7. Yuen PM, Chan NS, Yim SF, Chang AM. A randomised double blind comparison of Syntometrine and Syntocinon in the management of the third stage of labour. *Br J Obstet Gynaecol* 1995:102:377–80.
8. Hammar M, Boström K, Borgvall B. Comparison between the influence of methylergometrine and oxytocin on the incidence of retained placenta in the third stage of labour. *Gynecol Obstet Invest* 1990;30:91–3.
9. Soriano D, Dulitzki M, Schiff E, Barkai G, Mashiach S, Seidman DS. A prospective cohort study of oxytocin plus ergometrine compared with oxytocin alone for prevention of postpartum haemorrhage. *Br J Obstet Gynaecol* 1996;103:1068–73.
10. International Confederation of Midwives, International Federation of Gynaecologists and Obstetricians. Joint statement: management of the third stage of labour to prevent post-partum haemorrhage. *J Midwifery Womens Health* 2004;49:76–7.
11. World Health Organization. *WHO Recommendations for the Prevention of Postpartum Haemorrhage*. Geneva: WHO; 2007.
12. Leduc D, Senikas V, Lalonde AB, Ballerman C, Biringer A, Delaney M; Society of Obstetricians and Gynaecologists of Canada. Active management of the third stage of labour: prevention and treatment of postpartum haemorrhage. *J Obstet Gynaecol Can* 2009;31:980–93.
13. Royal College of Obstetricians and Gynaecologists. *Prevention and management of postpartum haemorrhage*. Green-top Guideline No. 52. RCOG: London; 2009 [http://www.rcog.org.uk/womens-health/clinical-guidance/prevention-and-management-postpartum-haemorrhage-green-top-52].
14. Davies GA, Tessier JL, Woodman MC, Lipson A, Hahn PM. Maternal hemodynamics after oxytocin bolus compared with infusion in the third

stage of labour: a randomized controlled trial. *Obstet Gynecol* 2005;105:294–9.

15. Thomas JS, Koh SH, Cooper GM. Haemodynamic effects of oxytocin given as i.v. bolus or infusion on women undergoing Caesarean section. *Br J Anaesth* 2007;98:116–9.

16. Baskett TF. A flux of the reds: evolution of active management of the third stage of labour. *J R Soc Med* 2000;93:489–93.

17. Hyashi RH, Castillo MS, Noah ML. Management of severe postpartum hemorrhage with a prostaglandin F2 alpha analogue. *Obstet Gynecol* 1984;63:806–8.

18. Oleen MA, Mariano JP. Controlling refractory atonic postpartum hemorrhage with Hemabate sterile solution. *Am J Obstet Gynecol* 1990;162:205–8.

19. Granström L, Ekman G, Ulmsten U. Intravenous infusion of 15 methyl-prostaglandin F2 alpha (Prostinfenem) in women with heavy post-partum hemorrhage. *Acta Obstet Gynecol Scand* 1989;68:365–7.

20. Boucher M, Nimrod CA, Tauragi GF, Meeker TA, Rennicks White RE, Varin J. Comparison of carbetocin and oxytocin for the prevention of postpartum haemorrhage following vaginal delivery: a double-blind randomized trial. *J Obstet Gynaecol Can* 2004;26:481–8.

21. Hofmeyr GJ, Walraven G, Gülmezoglu AM, Maholwana B, Alfirevic Z, Villar J. Misoprostol to treat postpartum haemorrhage: a systematic review. *BJOG* 2005;112:547–53.

22. Hofmeyr GJ, Gülmezoglu AM. Misoprostol for the prevention and treatment of postpartum haemorrhage. *Best Pract Res Clin Obstet Gynaecol* 2008;22:1025–41.

23. Weeks AD, Mirembe FM. The retained placenta – new insights into an old problem. *Eur J Obstet Gynecol Reprod Biol* 2002;102:109–10.

24. Weeks AD. The retained placenta. *Best Pract Res Clin Obstet Gynaecol* 2008;22:1103–17.

25. Bullarbo M, Tjugum J, Ekerhovd E. Sublingual nitroglycerin for management of retained placenta. *Int J Gynaecol Obstet* 2005;91:228–32.

26. Weeks AD, Alia G, Vernon G, Namayanja A, Gosakam R, Majeed T, et al. Umbilical vein oxytocin for the treatment of retained placenta (Release Study): a double-blind, randomised controlled trial. *Lancet* 2010;375:141–7.

27. Rogers MS, Yuen PM, Wong S. Avoiding manual removal of placenta: evaluation of intra-umbilical injection of uterotonics using the Pipingas technique for management of adherent placenta. *Acta Obstet Gynecol Scand* 2007;86:48–51.

6 Lower genital tract trauma

The cervix, vagina and perineum are vulnerable to trauma during descent and delivery of the baby. Indeed, some degree of trauma is almost inevitable, particularly in nulliparous women. In most cases the trauma is minor and full recovery can be expected, although perineal pain and superficial dyspareunia can persist for several weeks.[1] However, long-term studies have shown that uterovaginal prolapse and urinary and faecal incontinence are not uncommon following the stretching and tearing of the pelvic floor musculature and the enclosed branches of the pudendal nerve. In addition, a surprising amount of blood can be lost in a short period of time from lacerations of the perineum, vagina and cervix and this is a major risk factor for post-partum haemorrhage.[2] Knowledge of the predisposing factors and recognition and appropriate management of lower genital tract trauma are essential in the provision of safe obstetric care.

Factors associated with lower genital tract trauma include prolonged second stage of labour, early maternal pushing in the second stage of labour, macrosomia, persistent occipitoposterior position, assisted vaginal delivery (to a greater degree with forceps than with vacuum) and nulliparity.[3]

Classification

The perineum extends from the sub-pubic arch to the coccyx. The perineum is divided into two anatomical sites: the anterior urogenital and posterior anal triangles. Anterior perineal trauma involves the labia, anterior vaginal wall, periurethral and periclitoral regions. Posterior perineal injury includes the posterior vaginal wall, perineal muscles, anal sphincter and anorectal epithelium. This chapter reviews the following categories of trauma:

- episiotomy
- lacerations of vulva, vagina and cervix
- perineal tears
- haematomas.

EPISIOTOMY

While every effort should be made to deliver the fetal head over an intact perineum, episiotomy will be required in a number of cases. Reasons for episiotomy include the need to accelerate delivery for fetal distress and/or when the perineum is acting as an obstruction. It may also be required in assisted vaginal delivery when additional room is necessary for obstetric manoeuvres, such as those associated with assisted breech delivery, delivery of the second twin and shoulder dystocia.

Midline episiotomy is easier to repair and associated with less post-operative pain than a mediolateral episiotomy. However, the midline approach is more likely to extend into the anal sphincter and, for this reason, when episiotomy is indicated a mediolateral type is usually performed.

The principles of surgical repair of both types of episiotomy are similar and involve the following. First, it is very important to make a careful appraisal of the degree of damage following episiotomy. This may include a rectal examination to assess internal and external anal sphincter damage, which studies have shown to be frequently overlooked.[4,5]

The vascular tissues of the lower genital tract heal well, provided attention is paid to haemostasis and with careful but not excessively tight approximation of the tissue layers.

In general, use of the minimum possible amount of suture material and knots will limit tissue reaction and postoperative pain. This is usually best achieved with a continuous suture. A tapered, not cutting, needle is used with absorbable synthetic suture material: either polyglycolic acid (Dexon™ S; United States Surgical/TYCO Healthcare Group LP, New Haven, USA) or polyglactin 910 (Vicryl™; Ethicon/Johnson & Johnson, New Brunswick, USA) is suitable. However, these materials have delayed absorption which may lead to persistence and the need for removal of unabsorbed suture material some weeks after delivery. For this reason, the more rapidly absorbed 3/0 polyglactin 910 (Vicryl Rapide) is usually selected.[1]

The vagina and underlying fascia are closed with a continuous stitch starting 1 cm above the apex of the incision. If the tissues are very vascular, a locking stitch may be necessary. The suture is continued to the fourchette and held (Figure 6.1). Place the index finger into the wound, under the sutured vagina. This allows one to appreciate the extent and depth of the separation of the deep muscle layers, which should be reapproximated with either a continuous or individual sutures. In mediolateral episiotomies this may require a two-layer closure. The deep transverse and puborectalis muscles are brought together with individual sutures. The continuous vaginal suture, previously held at the fourchette,

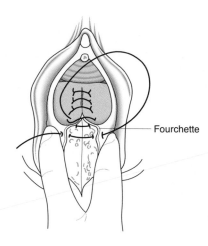

Fourchette

Figure 6.1 Episiotomy: repair of vaginal incision

is taken up again and directed through the vagina to the deeper tissues, then run down in a continuous side-to-side fashion approximately 1 cm from the edges of the vaginal skin (Figure 6.2). When the perineal apex of the episiotomy is reached, the suture is directed upwards as a continuous subcuticular suture back to the forchette, where it is tied (Figure 6.3). Sutures should not be put through the perineal skin, where they are irritating and painful and require removal.

At the end of the procedure, perform a rectal examination to confirm the integrity of the sphincters and to ensure that no sutures have been placed through the anorectal mucosa.

It is not uncommon, particularly with mediolateral episiotomies, for there to be considerable oozing of blood. Firm pressure applied with a pack for 2 minutes will often reduce this so that discrete bleeding points can be seen and sutured. It may be necessary to place a pack higher above the vaginal apex of the episiotomy during repair. If so, this pack must be tagged to ensure its removal at the end of the procedure. In any repair of lower genital tract trauma, there should be a swab and needle count at the end of the procedure. This is both good clinical practice and litigation risk management.

LACERATIONS OF THE VULVA, VAGINA AND CERVIX

In addition to perineal tears (page 67), individual lacerations of the vulva and vagina are common, while those of the cervix are less frequent.

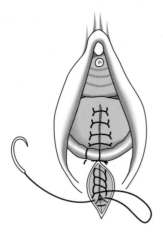 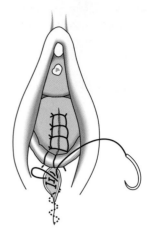

Figure 6.2 Episiotomy: repair of perineal muscles

Figure 6.3 Episiotomy: repair of perineal skin and subcutaneous tissues

Vulval lacerations

The most common vulval lacerations are those in the periurethral and periclitoral area. When episiotomy is not performed, the force from the descending head delivering over an intact perineum is transferred to the anterior perineal compartment and may result in periurethral and periclitoral tears. These are often quite superficial and, when the woman's hips are placed in the neutral position, the tears come together and require no sutures. If the tears are large and/or bleeding, a continuous subcuticular suture may be required. If stitching of periurethral lacerations is required, a Foley catheter should be inserted in the bladder to guide placement of the stitches.

Vaginal lacerations

Vaginal lacerations are common and may arise as an extension of the episiotomy. On other occasions the lacerations are independent and occur most commonly in the lower two-thirds of the vagina in the posterior sulci. Lacerations in the anterior sulci of the vagina are less common and tend to occur with more difficult access. Lacerations in the upper third of the vagina are not common and usually manifest as crescentic tears associated with rotational forceps delivery – a rare event nowadays.

Access to lacerations of the vagina can be difficult, particularly if there is persistent oozing. It is important to organise adequate assistance, lighting and retraction so that a properly conducted repair can be performed. Otherwise, the principles of suture are similar to those described for episiotomy (page 64). Usually, a continuous suture or, if there is excessive oozing, a locking suture is adequate. If the lacerations are extensive, and particularly if there is shearing and undermining of the underlying tissues, a vaginal pack should be placed for 18–24 hours following repair to avoid paravaginal haematoma formation. In these cases, a Foley catheter should be placed in the bladder.

Cervical lacerations

Cervical lacerations are not common. They are usually small, do not bleed and require no treatment. Occasionally, however, there may be considerable bleeding; in these cases, or if the laceration measures 3 cm or over, it should be repaired. One of the main difficulties is getting adequate exposure to inspect the entire cervix. This is best achieved with a pair of ring forceps. The anterior lip of the cervix is easily accessible and grasped with one ring forceps, while the second forceps is placed at approximately 2 o'clock. Remove the anterior (12 o'clock) forcep and pass it over to the 4 o'clock position; by repeating this 'leap-frog' technique, the entire circumference of the cervix can be inspected.

If a significant laceration is found, ring forceps are placed on each side and a continuous or locking suture is used to close the laceration and provide haemostasis. If, despite this treatment, the oozing continues, two ring forceps can be placed along each edge. The forceps can remain in place, with minimal disruption to the woman, for 2–4 hours before their removal.

Careful inspection of the upper vagina and cervix is always indicated in women with a steady trickle of blood postpartum associated with a well-contracted uterus. Good lighting and retraction are required for a complete assessment of the upper vagina and cervix. Appropriate use of the operating theatre, regional anaesthesia and assistance should be sought.

PERINEAL TEARS

The following classification of perineal tears has been proposed and is widely accepted. It allows comparisons of morbidity and different treatment techniques:[5]

- first degree: vaginal and perineal skin only
- second degree: division of skin and perineal muscles
- third degree: injury to the anal spincter complex, which may be one of three severities:
  - 3a: less than 50% of the external anal sphincter
  - 3b: more than 50% of the external anal sphincter
  - 3c: both the external and internal anal sphincter
- fourth degree: injury to the external and internal anal spincter and the anorectal mucosa.

The suture and repair of first- and second-degree perineal tears use the same principles as those for episiotomy repair.

The incidence of third- or fourth-degree tears varies from 0.5% to 5% of vaginal deliveries.[6,7] However, postpartum endo-anal ultrasound shows that almost one-third of women develop occult anal sphincter injury after their first vaginal delivery.[4,5] Therefore, after every delivery involving a lower genital tract laceration or tear, a thorough examination should take place looking specifically for trauma to the external anal sphincter and the internal anal sphincter. It is likely that the best chance of restoring long-term anal sphincter function is through the identification and careful repair of any anal sphincter damage. The following principles are relevant:

- Adequate regional anaesthesia is necessary to allow sufficient relaxation and analgesia to identify the disrupted tissues and perform the repair.
- Good lighting, positioning, equipment and assistance are essential.
- Close the anorectal mucosa with a gentle continuous suture of 3/0 Dexon or Vicryl (Figure 6.4a).
- Carefully identify the edges of the internal anal sphincter, which have a tendency to retract laterally to the anorectal mucosa. This should be repaired with interrupted stitches of the longer-lasting 3/0 polydioxanone (Maxon™, Tyco Healthcare UK Ltd, Gosport, Hampshire, UK) suture material (Figure 6.4b).
- After mediolateral episiotomy or a spontaneous third-degree tear, it is common for the external anal sphincter to be torn off to one side, rather than neatly in the midline. Often, one torn end of the sphincter will retract into a crater and have to be 'retrieved' using Allis forceps. Grasp both ends of the torn external anal sphincter with Allis forceps and clear the minimum amount of the adjacent connective tissue that will allow the ends of the endo-anal sphincter to be securely sutured together.

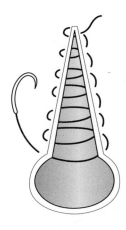
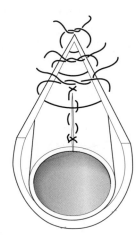

Figure 6.4a Third-/fourth-degree tear: suture of anorectal mucosa

Figure 6.4b Third-/fourth-degree tear: suture of internal anal sphincter

There are two accepted techniques for repair of a torn external anal sphincter, neither of which has been conclusively shown to be superior.[1,5,8,9] In the end-to-end technique, the torn ends are sutured together with two or three figure-of-eight stitches (Figure 6.5a). In the overlapping technique, at least two sutures are placed, as shown in Figure 6.5b, to achieve a 1.0–1.5 cm overlap of the muscle edges. The sutures are placed and held until all are in place and then tied down. Finally, two sutures are placed to anchor the free distal end of the underlying muscle to the overlapped edge above (Figure 6.5b). For both of these techniques, 3/0 polydioxanone/Maxon suture material is used. After the sphincter muscle has been repaired, the rest of the tissues are closed using the same principles as for episiotomy repair (page 64).

Broad-spectrum antibiotics should be given intraoperatively and for about 5 days postoperatively. Stool softeners and bulking agents should be given for 10–14 days following repair. Explanation and follow-up should be arranged, including emphasis on long-term pelvic floor exercises.

The potential for long-term morbidity, usually flatal and/or faecal incontinence, demands that repair of these injuries be performed by well-trained personnel. There is some evidence that appropriately structured training will improve results.[10]

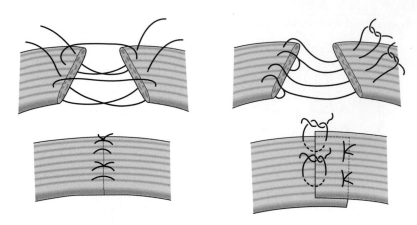

Figure 6.5a Repair of anal sphincter: end-to-end technique

Figure 6.5b Repair of anal sphincter: overlapping technique

HAEMATOMAS

Haematomas may be associated with assisted vaginal delivery, pudendal block and incomplete suturing of episiotomy or vaginal lacerations. In many cases there is no obvious trauma and the overlying vulvovaginal tissues are intact; indeed, the delivery may have been spontaneous and precipitate. The following types of haematoma are described: vulval, paravaginal and broad-ligament or supralevator haematomas.

Vulval haematomas

Vulval haematomas usually present soon after delivery as an acutely painful, tender, swollen area of the labium majus. The haematomas may be controlled with ice packs, analgesia and careful observation. If the haematomas enlarge, are greater than 5 cm and/or the pain is uncontrolled, they require incision and evacuation. The incision should be via the vagina if possible. Bleeding points should be oversewn with figure-of-eight sutures.

Paravaginal haematomas

Paravaginal haematomas are not visible externally and usually present with pain and restlessness in the postpartum hours. Inability to void is common and rectal tenesmus can occur. The diagnosis is confirmed by a gentle one-finger examination which reveals a tense, tender swelling protruding into and sometimes occluding the vagina. The treatment is incision and evacuation under regional or general anaesthesia. Often no discrete bleeding points are found, but any that are should be oversewn with figure-of-eight sutures. A Foley catheter should be placed in the bladder and the vagina tightly packed with gauze, lubricated with gel or cream to avoid abrasion and bleeding with removal of a dry pack. Others place the pack inside a sterile plastic bag to allow easier removal. In the case of a very capacious vagina, a blood pressure cuff can be put inside a sterile glove, placed in the vagina and inflated just above the systolic blood pressure.[11] Whichever technique is chosen, vaginal packing is the essential component in achieving haemostasis. The pack should be left in for 18–24 hours and the patient covered with broad-spectrum antibiotics.

Broad-ligament or supralevator haematomas

Broad-ligament or supralevator haematomas are uncommon but can occur if a blood vessel ruptures above the pelvic fascia. Blood loss can be considerable as the blood tracks between the leaves of the broad ligament and extends retroperitoneally – even as far as the kidneys. The clinical presentation can be of hypovolaemic shock and there may even be rupture into the peritoneal cavity. A broad-ligament haematoma may be felt on bimanual examination pushing the puerperal uterus to one side, and can track up the pelvic brim to the lateral abdominal wall in the iliac fossa. Ultrasound and magnetic resonance imaging can help to delineate and track the progression of these haematomas.

The initial management is conservative with intravenous crystalloid and blood if necessary, followed by tracking the stability or progress of the haematoma. If the haematoma increases and/or there are continuing signs of hypovolaemia, intervention is necessary. If available, angiographic embolisation of the involved branches of the internal iliac artery is the best approach, as this is the least invasive treatment and is usually successful. If this approach is not available, laparotomy is indicated with evacuation of the haematoma and ligation of bleeding points. At laparotomy, rupture of the lower uterine segment between the leaves of the broad ligament should be sought. Hysterectomy may be necessary.

References

1. Royal College of Obstetricians and Gynaecologists. *The management of third- and fourth-degree perineal tears*. Green-top Guideline No. 29. London: RCOG; 2007 [http://www.rcog.org.uk/womens-health/clinical-guidance/management-third-and-fourth-degree-perineal-tears-green-top-29].

2. Stones RW, Paterson CM, Saunders NJ. Risk factors for major obstetric haemorrhage. *Eur J Obstet Gynecol Reprod Biol* 1993;48:15–18.

3. Dudding TC, Vaizey CJ, Kamm MA. Obstetric anal sphincter injury: incidence, risk factors, and management. *Ann Surg* 2008;247:224–37.

4. Sultan AH, Kamm MA, Hudson CN, Thomas JM, Bartram CI. Anal sphincter disruption during vaginal delivery. *N Engl J Med* 1993;329:1905–11.

5. Sultan AH, Thakar R. Lower genital tract and anal sphincter trauma. *Best Pract Res Clin Obstet Gynaecol* 2002;16:99–115.

6. Samuelsson E, Ladfors L, Weinnerholm UB, Gåreberg B, Nyberg K, Hagberg H. Anal sphincter tears: prospective study of obstetric risk factors. *BJOG* 2000;107:926–31.

7. de Leeuw JW, Struijk PC, Vierhout ME, Wallenburg HC. Risk factors for third degree perineal ruptures during delivery. *BJOG* 2001;108:383–7.

8. Fitzpatrick M, Behan M, O'Connell PR, O'Herlihy C. A randomized clinical trial comparing primary overlap with approximation repair of third-degree obstetric tears. *Am J Obstet Gynecol* 2000;183:1220–4.

9. Farrell SA, Gilmour DT, Turnbull GK, Schmidt MH, Baskett TF, Flowerdew G, et al. Overlapping compared with end-to-end repair of third- and fourth-degree obstetric sphincter tears: a randomized controlled trial. *Obstet Gynecol* 2010;116:16–24.

10. Andrews V, Thakar R, Sultan AH. Outcome of obstetric anal sphincter injuries (OASIS) – role of structured management. *Int Urogynecol J* 2009;20:973–8.

11. Pinborg A, Bødker B, Høgdall C. Postpartum hematoma and vaginal packing with a blood pressure cuff. *Acta Obstet Gynecol Scand* 2000;79:887–9.

7 Induction of labour

Spontaneous onset of labour at term is the most desirable finale of pregnancy, heralding, as it usually does, the maturation of both fetal and maternal systems necessary for childbirth. Induction of labour is second best and this intervention is justified only for clear maternal, fetal or combined reasons. In induction of labour, uterine contractions are initiated by mechanical and/or pharmacological methods with the aim of achieving vaginal delivery. The options for induction of labour available in each centre should be discussed with the woman, including the possible success and failure rates and complications. The conditions for which induction is carried out will vary and depend on the medical or obstetric condition of the mother, the fetal condition, the knowledge and experience of the clinician, the willingness of the woman to undergo the procedure and the facilities available. Hence, the rates of induction of labour in the UK vary from 10% to 20%.

Indications and contraindications for induction of labour

There are several indications for induction of labour, the most common being:

- prolonged pregnancy (> 41 weeks)
- preterm prelabour rupture of membranes
- fetal growth restriction
- maternal conditions such as pre-eclampsia, diabetes, cholestasis or systemic lupus erythematosus
- abnormal antenatal fetal surveillance tests.

Contraindications to induction of labour include:

- maternal:
  - previous classical caesarean incision or multiple caesarean deliveries
  - infection, such as HIV or active genital herpes

o previous pregnancy/labour or delivery that resulted in anatomical or psychological trauma with concerns about labour and vaginal delivery in this pregnancy

● fetal:

o malpresentations such as face, brow or transverse/oblique lie

o fetal function tests that show severe compromise: preterminal cardiotocography (CTG) or absence or reversal of end diastolic umbilical artery blood flow

o placenta praevia or vasa praevia.

The potential benefits to the baby and the mother need to be assessed before undertaking induction of labour. There are relative indications, such as previous history of precipitate labour, suspicion of macrosomia and geographical isolation of the woman's home from the delivery unit. For such indications, induction carries no major benefit to the woman or the baby, hence one has to critically consider such cases on individual merit. Caution should be applied when inducing grand multiparous women and those with previous caesarean section, as there is an increased possibility of uterine rupture. Fetal death deserves special consideration, such as provision of an area isolated from the main labour ward where induction and labour can be carried out with sensitivity.

Complications of induction of labour

The risks of induction include prematurity if the gestation is uncertain, fetal compromise owing to overstimulation of the uterus, cord prolapse, chorioamnionitis, placental abruption, uterine rupture or failed induction leading to caesarean section. Failed induction is diagnosed when the woman does not go into labour, as manifested by an unchanged cervical score or when the cervix does not dilate to over 3 cm, so the woman does not enter the active phase of labour after a 12-hour period of artificial rupture of membranes and oxytocin infusion.[1] Failure to achieve vaginal delivery owing to poor progress in the active phase may be attributable to malposition or cephalopelvic disproportion. The prolonged use of oxytocin may be associated with neonatal jaundice. Oxytocin promotes water retention and, when given in large doses over a long time, may result in water intoxication.

Cervical priming

In cases where the cervix is unfavourable, the possibility of achieving a normal vaginal delivery can be enhanced by the use of prostaglandins or other methods to ripen the cervix before induction. The methods used for priming may initiate the onset of labour; this is often the case with the use of prostaglandins. The parity and period of gestation influence the cervical score and the readiness of the uterus to contract, which determines the success of induction of labour.[2] A favourable cervical score will more likely lead to easy induction and the establishment of labour, resulting in vaginal delivery (Table 7.1).

Table 7.1 Modified Bishop's score (reproduced with permission from Calder et al., 1974[3])				
Cervical parameter	Score			
	0	1	2	3
Position of cervix	Posterior	Middle	Anterior	–
Consistency of cervix	Firm	Medium	Soft	–
Station of presenting part (relative to ischial spines)	–3 cm	–2 cm	–1/0 cm	+1/+2 cm
Cervical dilatation	0 cm	1–2 cm	3–4 cm	> 4 cm
Cervical length	> 4 cm	3–4 cm	1–2 cm	< 1 cm

A score of 5–6 or more is considered favourable.

Medical or obstetric reasons should be the primary determinants for induction of labour. However, the state of the cervix and the likelihood of achieving vaginal delivery can help the timing of induction of labour. Thus, induction for soft indications such as poor obstetric history, psychosocial concern, previous rapid labour and relative geographical isolation have to be considered carefully based largely on the favourability of the cervix. Complications such as cord prolapse and placental abruption are rare, provided precautions are taken to rupture the membranes when the cervix is adequately dilated and the fetal head fits the brim of the pelvis. The National Institute for Health and Clincial Excellence (NICE) guidelines on induction of labour[2] recommend the use of prostaglandins for all women unless there is a special contraindication to the medication, such as the possibility of uterine hyperstimulation.

Studies on uterine activity in induced labour have suggested that about 60 000 kilopascals of total uterine activity is needed to induce and achieve full dilatation in a primigravid woman with an unfavourable cervix, compared with about 32 000 kilopascals if she has a favourable cervical score. In a multigravid woman, the total uterine activity needed with a poor cervical score is about 32 000 kilopascals and 16 000 kilopascals when she has a favourable cervical score.[4] Therefore, parity and the state of the cervix are the key prognostic factors for successful induction.

The cervix can be primed using mechanical[5] or pharmacological methods[2] before induction of labour.

MECHANICAL METHODS

Membrane sweeping/stripping

Membrane sweeping/stripping is an accepted method of priming the cervix. The membranes can be stripped from the internal os and the lower uterine segment by passing a finger through the cervix and sweeping the membranes around the presenting part. The mechanism of action is the release of prostaglandins as a result of the inflammation caused over the following few days and the possible action of phospholipase A2 in the membranes, which causes the synthesis and release of endogenous prostaglandin to ripen the cervix. Some women may find this procedure unacceptable and uncomfortable. Women should be advised of the discomfort they might experience from the examination, subsequent painful uterine contractions and a probable blood-stained discharge for the next 2–3 days, and should be asked to report to the hospital if their membranes rupture, if there is frank bleeding or if uterine contractions become more frequent and regular. A systematic review consisting of 21 studies suggests that membrane sweeping allows fewer women to be induced within 1 week, as some go into labour over the few days following the procedure.[6] Many hospitals in the UK use membrane sweeping as a standard method and offer it to women at 41 weeks or 41[+3] weeks of pregnancy. Available evidence suggests that there is no increased risk of infection to the mother or the neonate. Apart from the discomfort of the examination, membrane sweeping is a simple procedure, although it is usually effective only if the cervix is sufficiently patulous to allow entry of the finger through the internal os.

Mechanical dilatation

The seaweed *Laminaria japonica*, in a dehydrated form, is placed within the cervical canal. The seaweed imbibes water and expands, causing mechanical dilatation. Based on a similar principle, a synthetic polyvinyl sponge with magnesium sulphate (Lamicel®, Medtronic Xomed, Inc., Jacksonville, FL, USA) can be used for cervical ripening. The latter approach is more sterile and is likely to give rise to less infection. Usually, such mechanical dilators are inserted 12 hours before the planned induction; that is, the previous night. Induction is then carried out the next morning by rupture of membranes and oxytocin infusion.[7]

Catheters

A Foley catheter and specially designed double-balloon catheters are used to ripen the cervix in some centres. The catheter is passed through the cervical canal and the balloon inflated with 30–50 ml saline. The catheter is left in place until it drops out, or for 12–24 hours.[5] The use of a balloon followed by oxytocin is recommended by the World Health Organization (WHO) for units where prostaglandins are not available.[8]

Amniotomy

In the past, amniotomy was used to prime the cervix and to induce labour. About 80–90% of women go into labour within 24 hours of rupture of membranes. However, the incidence of infection is slightly increased and the induction-to-delivery interval is longer compared with rupture of membranes with simultaneous use of oxytocin infusion.

Mechanical methods may be useful if prostaglandins are not available, are contraindicated or if there is concern about potential uterine hyper-stimulation. Prostaglandins need refrigeration, except for misoprostol, which is a prostaglandin E1 compound and which is increasingly used in developing countries, as recommended by WHO.[8]

PHARMACOLOGICAL METHODS

Prostaglandins

Although oral prostaglandin is more effective than placebo in reducing the caesarean section rate with induction of labour, the same effectiveness can be achieved by priming the cervix using vaginal or intracervical prostaglandin. The gastrointestinal adverse effects are markedly increased with oral prostaglandins, so they are not used for induction of labour. Intravenous prostaglandins, which were used a few decades ago, are contraindicated because of increased uterine hyper-stimulation, gastrointestinal adverse effects and no better success rate compared with intravenous oxytocin or vaginal prostaglandins.[2]

Extra-amniotic prostaglandin reduces the requirement for oxytocin augmentation compared with placebo. However, vaginal prostaglandin has a similar or better outcome and hence extra-amniotic prostaglandin E2 (PGE2), which is an invasive procedure, is rarely used. Intracervical PGE2 is less effective compared with vaginal PGE2 in achieving vaginal birth within 24 hours in women with an unfavourable cervix. In women with a favourable cervix, maternal and fetal outcomes are similar whether intra-cervical or vaginal prostaglandins are used.

Hence, the recommendation is to use vaginal and not intracervical prostaglandins.[2]

Oxytocin infusion

The use of oxytocin is not recommended in women with an unfavourable cervix and intact membranes as it is less effective than vaginal PGE2 in improving the cervical score or reducing the caesarean section rate. In those with an unfavourable cervix but ruptured membranes, intravenous oxytocin is less effective compared with PGE2 in effecting vaginal birth within 24 hours. Similarly, in women with a favourable cervix, intravenous oxytocin in not as effective compared with vaginal prostaglandin in achieving vaginal delivery within 24 hours. Hence, intravenous oxytocin alone is not used for induction of labour.

Amniotomy and use of oxytocin in women with an unfavourable cervix, compared with PGE2 vaginally, has not been proved to be more effective. Once amniotomy is performed, a woman is committed to delivery and hence it is better to use PGE2 vaginally in women with poor cervical scores. In women with favourable cervical scores, oxytocin infusion and amniotomy can be effective but reduces the woman's ability to move around in the early part of induction. Hence, amniotomy and oxytocin is generally not used as primary method of induction even in women with a good cervical score, but it is of value in women with contraindications to the use of vaginal PGE2.

Misoprostol

Misoprostol is increasingly used in developing countries, although it is not licensed for use for induction of labour. The routes of administration used are oral, vaginal and sublingual and the doses used are 50 micrograms or 25 micrograms. These doses can be achieved only by using a pill cutter and trying to reduce the 100 microgram or 200 microgram tablets. This makes accurate dosage administration more difficult. Oral misoprostol 100 micrograms is more likely to be associated with meconium-stained liquor compared with oxytocin infusion. Both 50 micrograms and 100 micrograms of misoprostol have similar maternal and fetal outcome.

NICE recommends that misoprostol not be used for induction of labour as it is not licensed for this purpose.[2] When misoprostol is used for clinical trial purposes and in centres where vaginal PGE2 is not available, the oral dose of 50 micrograms is recommended, as higher doses are associated with uterine hyperstimulation. Vaginally, 25 micrograms of misoprostol is acceptable, although it is not superior to vaginal

PGE2. Although successful induction of labour is achieved using 25 micrograms of misoprostol vaginally, there is a higher incidence of uterine hyperstimulation and meconium staining of amniotic fluid. WHO supports the use of misoprostol for induction of labour.[8] The recommended dose is oral misoprostol 25 micrograms 2-hourly or vaginal misoprostol 25 micrograms 6-hourly. This approach is contraindicated for women with a previous caesarean section or other uterine scar.[8]

Other medications

Estrogens, hyaluronidase and corticosteroids have been tried for induction of labour, but without benefit. Vaginal glyceryl trinitrate and nitric oxide donors have been compared with vaginal PGE2 as induction agents. They reduce uterine hyperstimulation but are less effective than PGE2, have significant adverse effects and are not recommended for induction of labour.

Herbal supplementation, acupuncture, homeopathy, castor oil, hot bath and enema, breast stimulation and sexual intercourse have all been tried for induction of labour, but the value of these methods is not proven.

Monitoring the fetus during induction of labour

The process of induction of labour aims to produce uterine contractions, which can cause reduction of placental perfusion as well as cord compression. It is ideal to have 45 minutes to 1 hour of CTG tracing before induction and for a period of 1 hour after the introduction of vaginal prostaglandin in case there is rapid absorption and uterine hyperstimulation. The absorption of prostaglandin is dependent on moisture content, pH, temperature and the presence of infection in the vagina. If the CTG trace is normal before and for about 1 hour after the insertion of the prostaglandin, the woman can ambulate and be monitored when regular contractions begin.

Information provided to women

It is important for health professionals to explain the reason for induction, including when, where and how the induction will be carried out. The method of fetal and maternal surveillance and pain relief offered should be explained. If there are any alternatives to induction of labour, or the possibility of postponement, they should be discussed. Women may ask for different methods of induction and a clear explanation should be offered for the method chosen.

Induction for specific circumstances

INDUCTION OF LABOUR IN WOMEN AT OR BEYOND TERM

The epidemiological evidence suggests that there is an increased risk for mother and baby as the pregnancy continues beyond 40 weeks, and a further increased risk after 42 weeks. The first large randomised trial found an advantage to the fetus and mother of induction of labour at between 41 and 42 weeks of gestation.[9] Twenty-two controlled trials have evaluated the benefits of inducing labour at 37–40 weeks, 41 completed weeks and 42 completed weeks.[10] Eight perinatal deaths occurred in 12 trials, all in the expectant group after 41 weeks. WHO does not recommend induction at less than 41 weeks with an uncomplicated pregnancy or in those who are unsure of dates; the current recommendation is to offer induction of labour in uncomplicated pregnancies after 41 completed weeks.[8] The exact timing should be based on the woman's preferences and the availability of beds in the local unit. In cases where the woman would like to continue with her pregnancy beyond 42 weeks, antenatal fetal testing in the form of twice-weekly CTG and maximum amniotic pool depth should be carried out.[2]

PRETERM PRELABOUR RUPTURE OF MEMBRANES

Preterm prelabour rupture of membranes, at less than 37 weeks of gestation, occurs in about 3% of the obstetric population. Evidence suggests that induction of labour is best avoided in women at less than 34 weeks of gestation unless additional complications are identified, such as fetal compromise or possible chorioamnionitis. After 34 weeks of gestation, the risks should be discussed with the woman: sepsis, the possible need for caesarean section and preterm birth in the context of available neonatal intensive care facilities. It is usual to recommend induction of labour in these cases. In women with prelabour rupture of membranes at term – that is, beyond 37 weeks of gestation – induction of labour should be offered with vaginal PGE2 or with oxytocin infusion.

PREVIOUS CAESAREAN SECTION

Previous caesarean section is not a contraindication to induction of labour. If induction is needed in a woman with previous caesarean section for obstetric reasons, artificial rupture of membranes, oxytocin infusion or PGE2 vaginal pessaries can be used. However, the woman must be informed that the use of oxytocin increases the risk of uterine rupture and that PGE2 further increases that risk.[11] Although the risk of uterine rupture is small, it is significantly increased (two- to three-fold) with the use of oxytocic drugs. This must be clearly relayed to the woman. This is discussed further in chapter 14.

MATERNAL REQUEST FOR INDUCTION OF LABOUR

At times, women request induction of labour for convenience for the family rather than for a medical indication. This may be considered at or after 40 weeks of gestation, but the parity and cervical score should be carefully assessed to avoid the possibility of failed induction and caesarean section.

STABILISING INDUCTION

Women with unstable, oblique or transverse lie at term may run the risk of cord prolapse or obstructed labour should they start spontaneous labour or have ruptured membranes. In the absence of contraindications to vaginal delivery or external cephalic version, stabilising induction at or near 40 weeks may be a suitable option in those with a favourable cervix. The woman and her partner should be advised of the risk of cord prolapse and the chance of the fetus reverting to a transverse or oblique lie. If the woman accepts stabilising induction, external cephalic version is carried out. The operator holds the head just above the pelvic brim, starts an oxytocin infusion and, when uterine contractions stabilise the head at the pelvic brim, the membranes are ruptured with slow release of amniotic fluid to settle the head further. The mother and fetus should be carefully monitored until such time as one is confident that the lie and presentation have stabilised.

FETAL DEATH OR FETUS WITH LETHAL MALFORMATION

Induction of labour for fetal death or severe anomaly can be emotionally devastating for the couple. This is compounded by the fact that the duration of the induction is unpredictable, as the induction often takes place at an earlier gestation when the cervix may not be favourable and the uterus less sensitive to the oxytocics. Emotional support, privacy and care by specially trained midwives are of great value. The specialist should be involved in the woman's care. The choice of immediate or delayed induction may be offered, except in cases where the membranes have ruptured, there is bleeding or there are signs of infection. Available evidence recommends the use of vaginal or oral misoprostol for induction of labour.[8] The chance of uterine rupture with induction close to term in women with a previous caesarean should be kept in mind.[2] The RCOG has issued specific detailed guidelines for management of fetal death:

mifepristone 200 mg, followed 12–24 hours later by misoprostol 100 micrograms 6-hourly before 26 weeks, or 25–50 micrograms 4-hourly after 27 weeks.[12] Gemeprost is equally effective but costs more and is not available in all centres. PGE2 can be used at term.

Conclusion

The philosophy surrounding induction of labour is changing. Induction of labour has potential complications and should be undertaken only when there are clear benefits to the mother and/or the fetus. In addition to the medical or obstetric condition for which the induction is undertaken, due consideration should be given to parity, gestation, cervical score and the presence or absence of intact fetal membranes. Iatrogenic hazards of unexpected prematurity, cord prolapse, uterine hyperstimulation, uterine rupture and iatrogenic fetal hypoxia and neonatal morbidity should be avoided. The staff and facilities should be optimal to monitor the mother and fetus and to look after the newborn. Women who receive oxytocics have a real risk of sudden uterine hyperstimulation and fetal compromise within a short period, and a midwife should be at the bedside when the mother is in active labour. Induction of labour should take place in a unit where there is ready recourse to caesarean section. WHO is keen to drive the concept that failed induction, with intact membranes, does not necessarily equate to immediate delivery by caesarean section; if adopted, this may reduce the number of unnecessary caesarean sections.[8]

References

1. Arulkumaran S, Gibb DM, TambyRaja RL, Heng SH, Ratnam SS. Failed induction of labour. *Aust N Z J Obstet Gynaecol* 1985;25:190–3.
2. National Collaborating Centre for Women's and Children's Health, National Institute for Health and Clinical Excellence. *Induction of labour. Clinical Guideline*. London: RCOG Press; 2008 [http://guidance.nice.org.uk/CG70].
3. Calder AA, Embrey MP, Hillier K. Extra-amniotic prostaglandin E2 for the induction of labour at term. *J Obstet Gynaecol Br Commonw* 1974;81:39–46.
4. Arulkumaran S, Gibb DM, Ratnam SS, Lun KC, Heng SH. Total uterine activity in induced labour – an index of cervical and pelvic tissue resistance. *Br J Obstet Gynaecol* 1985;92:693–7.
5. Boulvain M, Kelly A, Lohse C, Stan CM, Irion O. Mechanical methods for induction of labour. *Cochrane Database Syst Rev* 2001;(4):CD001233.
6. Boulvain M, Stan CM, Irion O. Membrane sweeping for induction of labour. *Cochrane Database Syst Rev* 2005;(1):CD000451.
7. Chua S, Arulkumaran S, Vanaia K, Ratnam SS. Preinduction cervical ripening: prostaglandin E2 gel vs hygroscopic mechanical dilator. *J Obstet Gynecol Res* 1997;23:171–7.

8. World Health Organization, Department of Reproductive Health and Research. *WHO recommendations for induction of labour.* Geneva: WHO; 2011 [http://www.who.int/reproductivehealth/publications/maternal_perinatal_health/9789241501156/en/].

9. Hannah ME, Hannah WJ, Hellmann J, Hewson S, Milner R, Willan A. Induction of labor as compared with serial antenatal monitoring in post-term pregnancy. A randomized controlled trial. The Canadian Multicenter Post-term Pregnancy Trial Group. *N Engl J Med* 1992;326;1587–92.

10. Gülmezoglu AM, Crowther CA, Middleton P. Induction of labour for improving birth outcomes for women at or beyond term. *Cochrane Database Syst Rev* 2006;(4):CD004945.

11. McDonagh MS, Osterweil P, Guise JM. The benefits and risks of inducing labour in patients with prior caesarean delivery: a systematic review. *BJOG* 2005;112:1007–15.

12. Royal College of Obstetricians and Gynaecologists. *Late intrauterine fetal death and stillbirth.* Green-top Guideline No. 55. London: RCOG; 2010 [http://www.rcog.org.uk/womens-health/clinical-guidance/late-intrauterine-fetal-death-and-stillbirth-green-top-55].

8   Preterm labour and prelabour rupture of membranes

Preterm birth is defined as delivery before the 37th completed week of gestation; there is no definitive definition of the lower limit. The World Health Organization considers a fetus over 22 weeks of gestation at the limit of viability. In the absence of known gestation, a birth weight of 500 g has been considered potentially compatible with life. Available data show the mortality rate to be high up to 24 weeks of gestation; therefore, many countries, including the UK, consider 24 weeks as the cut-off point for fetal viability.[1,2] Births between 24 and 37 weeks of gestation account for 5–12% of total deliveries. Rates of preterm birth differ from country to country and from region to region within countries, depending on the definitions used. Although there are a relatively small number of preterm births, they contribute to nearly 70% of all perinatal deaths.[3] Mortality and neurological morbidity are greater at early gestations and much lower after 28 weeks of gestation.[4] The long-term handicap may manifest as blindness, deafness or cerebral palsy, in addition to chronic respiratory disorders. The majority of women who present with uterine contractions in the preterm period do not progress to established labour. Hence, more women than necessary may be treated with tocolytics to prevent or abolish uterine contractions and with corticosteroids to enhance fetal lung maturity. Management varies based on whether the woman presents in preterm labour with or without prelabour rupture of membranes. This chapter covers preterm labour and prelabour rupture of membranes preterm and at term.

Risk factors for preterm delivery

Preterm labour and delivery are associated with several conditions related to pregnancy or the reproductive tract:

- previous history of preterm birth
- multiple pregnancies
- prelabour rupture of membranes
- pre-eclampsia

- fetal growth restriction
- previous conisation of the cervix
- acquired or congenital malformations of the uterus, such as uterine fibroids, bicornuate uterus.

Medical conditions unrelated to the reproductive tract have been postulated to be associated with preterm labour, although the link appears to be weak:

- urinary tract infection
- pyrexia
- gingivitis[5]
- sickle cell disease.[6]

In general, one-third of preterm births before 34 weeks of gestation are iatrogenic – that is, there is a medical indication to intervene and deliver the baby[7] – one-third are a result of prelabour rupture of membranes and in one-third the cause is unknown, but possibly attributable to infection. Infection should be excluded if preterm labour is to be suppressed with a view to continuing the pregnancy.

Prediction and prevention of preterm labour

The consequences for the newborn, the parents and families are profound when a baby is delivered preterm, particularly for those born before 26 weeks of gestation. In addition, the short- and long-term costs to the health service are considerable, and probably exceed what that individual can earn in a lifetime. Because of the high morbidity and mortality associated with preterm birth, it is important to try and predict and prevent preterm labour.

Bacterial vaginosis has been considered a potential factor in triggering preterm labour. The infection can start in early gestation, at 14 or 15 weeks, although the woman might present later, at 19–24 weeks, with slow dilatation of the cervix and preterm labour. To prevent such early births, the biochemical clock has to be stopped before the anatomical changes take place. Studies are contradictory about screening for and treating bacterial vaginosis routinely or only in women with a previous history of late fetal loss or preterm birth. One study showed a reduction in the incidence of preterm birth when treated with oral clindamycin,[8] while others showed a tendency to increased incidence of preterm birth when treated with metronidazole.[9,10]

Progesterone has been shown to be beneficial in delaying preterm delivery in women who have shortening of the cervix on ultrasound examination.[11,12] Progesterone can be administered as a vaginal pessary and is used in women who have previous preterm birth or those who have threatened preterm labour.

Case selection for early prophylactic cerclage is difficult. Routine screening for cervical length (less than 1.5 cm) and applying prophylactic cervical cerclage is not effective,[13] although it may be of benefit in women with a previous preterm birth and a short cervix of less than 2.5 cm.[14] Cervical cerclage may be effective in those with a previous history of painless cervical dilatation at 22–26 weeks of gestation that progressed to preterm labour and delivery. Studies on multiple pregnancies have shown that prophylactic cervical cerclage has no value.

Emergency cerclage, performed after cervical dilatation has been observed, is controversial. Some women may have had slow cervical dilatation owing to infection, in which case the mechanical solution of cerclage for a biochemical problem of infection and release of prostaglandins will not be effective. When the cervix dilates to 4–6 cm, attempts to reduce the membranes and apply cervical cerclage are fraught with difficulty because the membranes in these cases tend to bulge with tension. Emergency cerclage has a high failure rate. There is also the possibility of subclinical intrauterine infection in these cases. Thus, emergency cerclage is best performed rarely and on a case-by-case basis.

Multiple pregnancies are a clearly identified cause of preterm delivery, as outlined in chapter 12. The undisciplined application of assisted reproductive technology has contributed to multiple pregnancies becoming the cause of almost 25% of all preterm births below 32 weeks of gestation. As a result, many countries have regulated single-embryo transfer with in vitro fertilisation in an attempt to reduce the mortality and morbidity of preterm delivery in multiple pregnancies. In cases where there are three or more embryos, selective fetal reduction is practised in some centres to prevent preterm birth.

Transvaginal ultrasound to examine the cervix is increasingly used to assess asymptomatic women in whom it has been shown that the chance of delivering preterm increases six-fold if the cervical length is below the 10th centile (less than 2.5 cm) between 22 and 24 weeks of gestation.[15] In symptomatic women with a singleton pregnancy, the risk of delivery within 7 days is 40–50% if the length of the cervix is less than 15 mm. The addition of the fetal fibronectin test will enhance the sensitivity and specificity of these predictions (see page 89).

Clinical presentation and investigation of preterm labour

HISTORY

The following symptoms may suggest preterm labour:

- regular uterine contractions (over six per hour)
- lower abdominal pain/cramps
- low-back ache/pelvic pressure of recent onset
- mucous or blood-stained show
- ruptured membranes.

The differential diagnosis includes intestinal or urinary colic. Continuous pain suggests the possibility of abruption or another pathology such as red degeneration in a fibroid. Abruption can give rise to preterm labour and should be excluded before conservative management. Previous history of late fetal loss or spontaneous preterm birth, together with the above symptoms, is a strong suggestion of preterm labour.

EXAMINATION

Pulse, blood pressure, temperature and respiratory rate will help to exclude possible infection or abruption. Uterine tenderness owing to abruption or infection should be excluded.

The lie and presentation of the fetus will influence the mode of delivery and this should be established clinically or, if needed, by ultrasound. Fetal presentation above the pelvic brim with a long and closed cervix on ultrasound or digital examination is less likely to be associated with progressive preterm labour.

Speculum examination should be carried out to determine the length and dilatation of the cervix and to rule out ruptured membranes or bleeding. In the absence of ruptured membranes, a gentle vaginal examination can be performed to establish the cervical status.

INVESTIGATIONS

Based on the clinical presentation, some or all of the following investigations should be carried out:

- Full blood count, as a baseline measure and to look for elevated white cell count.
- C-reactive protein: a significant rise would indicate infection.
- High vaginal swab to rule out pathogens.

- Low vaginal swab with a sweep of the perineum and the anal canal to identify group B streptococcus.

- Mid-stream sample of urine for microscopy and culture.

- Ultrasound examination to confirm the fetal lie and presentation. The presence of amniotic fluid below the presenting part when the mother is in the semi-prone position should exclude leakage of fluid. Marked oligohydramnios is suggestive of ruptured membranes.

- Fetal weight can be estimated using fetal biometry of abdominal circumference, femur length and head circumference.

- Ultrasound to determine the length of the cervix.

- Fetal fibronectin is a glycoprotein produced by the chorionic membranes which acts as a tissue glue to bind the membranes to the decidua. It is found in cervical/vaginal secretions at less than 22 weeks of gestation and before labour, but normally not between 24 and 34 weeks of gestation unless there is disruption of the membranes from the deciduas, which may presage preterm labour. The swab for the test is taken from the posterior vaginal fornix with an unlubricated speculum (lubricants can cause a false-negative result). No vaginal examination or transvaginal ultrasound should be performed in the 24 hours before the swab is taken. False-positive results can be found in the presence of blood, amniotic fluid and semen. In a review of 40 studies involving more than 11 000 women with symptoms of preterm labour, those with a negative test had a less than 2% chance of delivery within 7–14 days, whereas 20–30% of women with a positive test delivered within 7–14 days.[16] In most studies, only 10–20% of women with symptoms of preterm labour will have a positive test. Thus, there is clear value in this test as a guide to subsequent clinical management, such as admission to hospital and/or the administration of corticosteroids or tocolytic drugs.

Management of preterm labour

GENERAL MANAGEMENT

The neonatal unit should be informed of the possible need for resources for a preterm neonate. If the unit is not equipped to provide such care, in utero transfer should be considered and arranged.

Provide adequate hydration and nutrition for the mother, pain relief as necessary and appropriate counselling and support to allay the anxiety of parents and family. The mother and her partner should be counselled regarding the possible consequences of delivery at that gestation.

Team coordination between the obstetricians, neonatologists and midwives is essential to manage such cases, with the obstetrician taking the lead. An experienced paediatrician should be present at the delivery. A clear plan of action should be written in the notes, including the management of labour: whether the mother will have tocolysis, steroids and antibiotics, whether the fetus will be monitored and the mode of delivery.

SPECIFIC MANAGEMENT

Steroids should be given to promote fetal lung maturity. Steroids promote type II pneumocytes to release surfactant into the lungs, which reduces surface tension and hence lessens the incidence of hyaline membrane disease and respiratory distress syndrome. To administer the steroids, preterm uterine contractions may need to be suppressed for a period of 24–48 hours. This may be achieved by administration of a suitable tocolytic agent. Antibiotics should be given if there is suspicion of infection. The use of steroids, tocolytic agents and antibiotics is discussed below.

Tocolytics

Tocolysis for prevention of preterm birth is used widely, despite no clear advantage in improving perinatal outcome. The main rationale for tocolysis is short-term delay of labour to allow maternal transfer and/or completion of the course of corticosteroids.

Until recently, ritodrine, a beta 2-receptor agonist that relaxes uterine smooth muscle, was used extensively. Isoxsuprine, terbutaline, salbutamol, magnesium sulphate, nifedipine, indometacin and atosiban are used in different centres. These medications can have severe adverse effects and it is best not to use them in combination. A review of 17 trials showed that beta-agonists, indometacin and atosiban were associated with a significant reduction of births within 24 hours, 48 hours or up to 7 days, but magnesium sulphate was ineffective.[17] None of the tocolytic drugs was able to reduce the number of births before 30, 32 or 37 weeks of gestation.[18]

Furthermore, the use of a tocolytic drug alone to prevent preterm birth was not associated with a reduction in neonatal morbidity or mortality. There is some concern about an increase in deaths in the first year of life associated with atosiban compared with placebo,[19] which may be attributable to the fetal vasopressin receptor blockade by atosiban and its impact on renal and lung development. However, long-term studies are needed to confirm or refute this. The composite outcome study of perinatal deaths, chronic lung disease, necrotising enterocolitis and significant intraventricular haemorrhage showed better (borderline significant) outcome with glyceryl trinitrate skin patches compared with placebo.[20]

Nifedipine and atosiban have comparable efficacy in prolonging pregnancy up to 7 days. Compared with betamimetic drugs, nifedipine appears to have a better neonatal outcome, but long-term follow-up data are needed to confirm this. Compared with betamimetics, which have a high incidence of adverse effects, nifedipine, atosiban and cyclo-oxygenase inhibitors have fewer adverse effects, and most of the major adverse effects observed were in women taking multiple medications.[20]

Calcium channel blockers (nifedipine) appear to have a beneficial effect on reducing neonatal respiratory distress, necrotising enterocolitis and intraventricular haemorrhage compared with other medications. However, there is no difference in the number of stillbirths or neonatal deaths. Magnesium sulphate does not appear to reduce the incidence of preterm birth,[20] but it does reduce the risk of cerebral palsy[21] and it may be useful for women to have 24 hours of magnesium sulphate if they are at risk of preterm birth.[20]

Glyceryl trinitrate is used in the form of skin patches of 10 mg initially and, if required, a further 10 mg 2 hours later with a maximum total dose of 20 mg over 24 hours. The woman should be warned of flushing, occasional giddiness and headache caused by peripheral vasodilatation.

Indometacin is given in a dose of 1–3 mg/kg body weight of the mother. It should be avoided after 32 weeks of gestation because continued use is associated with renal and pulmonary artery vasoconstriction leading to oligohydramnios and pulmonary hypertension.

Nifedipine is given orally as a 20 mg dose followed by 10–20 mg three to four times a day. Based on uterine activity, this can be continued for up to 48 hours. A total dose over 60 mg is associated with a four-fold increase in the number of adverse effects. In many units nifedipine is the tocolytic of choice.

Atosiban is given as a 6.75 mg slow intravenous bolus dose followed by an infusion of 18 mg/hour over 3 hours. The dosage is subsequently reduced to 6 mg/hour for up to 48 hours, or a maximum of 330 mg.

In terms of cost, the atosiban regimen costs £494 for a 48-hour treatment cycle compared with £1 for nifedipine and £50 for ritodrine.[20]

Based on the available evidence, it is reasonable to use tocolysis for short-term prolongation of pregnancy to enable corticosteroids to be given for lung maturity or the woman to be transferred to another hospital. Caution must be exercised not to prolong a pregnancy where it is contraindicated, such as in suspected cases of infection, chorioamnionitis or fetal growth restriction with signs of fetal compromise.

The efficacy of tocolytic drugs in multiple pregnancies is unclear, but they should be used to allow administration of corticosteroids to achieve fetal lung maturity. Maintenance tocolytic therapy is not recommended as it is ineffective and may mask subclinical infection.

Antenatal corticosteroids

Corticosteroids reduce neonatal morbidity and mortality in the preterm period owing to a significant reduction in rates of respiratory distress syndrome and intraventricular haemorrhage. There are no major adverse effects attributable to the administration of corticosteroids alone, and they should be given to any woman with threatened preterm delivery between 24 and 34 weeks of gestation.[22] The impact of the medication is seen after 24 hours and up to 7 days after administration of the second dose. Although the maximal impact is after 24 hours, there is some effect even if the baby is delivered within 24 hours of giving corticosteroids, and it is therefore best to give corticosteroids as soon as possible.[22]

Current knowledge indicates that there are no significant short-term maternal or fetal adverse effects of corticosteroids and, although there is a debate about long-term adverse effects, there appear to be no adverse neurological or cognitive sequelae.[23] The effect of multiple doses of corticosteroids is not known and is the subject of study. Corticosteroids suppress the immune system, hence one should be cautious and avoid giving corticosteroid therapy in women with systemic infection such as sepsis or tuberculosis. When there is overt chorioamnionitis, corticosteroids can be given, but if there are maternal or fetal concerns there should be no delay in delivery.

There is no place for prophylactic corticosteroid therapy for women with a previous history of preterm birth or in women with multiple pregnancies. There is no need to give a double dose of corticosteroids in multiple pregnancies. In women with diabetes mellitus, the adminis-tration of corticosteroids is not contraindicated, but the blood glucose should be closely monitored and, if necessary, additional insulin should be given according to protocol. In fetuses with fetal growth restriction between 24 and 34 weeks of gestation, it may be best to offer a single course of antenatal corticosteroids. In many centres corticosteroids are given to women who are to be delivered because of medical reasons, or in women who go into spontaneous labour before 34 weeks of gestation.

There has been some debate about whether the corticosteroid administered should be betamethasone or dexamethasone, but current evidence supports two doses of betamethasone 12 mg intramuscularly, 24 hours apart. Whether the antenatal course of corticosteroids should be repeated is not clear, as there is some concern about reduction in birth weight and head circumference. Hence, weekly administration is not recommended, but a rescue course of the same dose may be considered with caution when the steroids were given at less than 26 weeks of gestation.

Antibiotics

Although antibiotics were found to prolong pregnancy and reduce the incidence of maternal infection, there was no significant reduction in neonatal deaths or respiratory problems.[24] The 7-year follow-up of one of the trials of preterm labour in women with intact membranes has suggested a slightly increased incidence of neurological disorders in those who received antibiotics compared with the placebo group.[25] Based on these findings, routine administration of antibiotics is not recommended in those with preterm labour and intact membranes.

Preterm prelabour rupture of membranes

The incidence of preterm prelabour rupture of membranes (PPROM) is about 2%, but it contributes to 40% of preterm deliveries.[26] One-third of women with PPROM may have occult infection. Studies that looked for infection via amniocentesis suggest that either infecting organisms or metabolites following infection can be detected in 30–35% of women with PPROM.[27]

HISTORY

There may be continuous dribbling of fluid with dampness of sanitary pads. Women can usually distinguish between this and leakage from the bladder.

CLINICAL EXAMINATION

General observations of maternal pulse, blood pressure, temperature, respiratory rate and uterine tenderness should be performed. Abdominal examination should be performed to assess fundal height, lie and presentation and to exclude uterine tenderness. Fetal heart rate should be recorded.

Vaginal digital examination is avoided for the fear of introducing infection in cases where rupture of membranes is suspected. Speculum examination helps to confirm pooling of liquor in the posterior fornix. In cases of doubt, liquor emerging through the cervical os when the mother coughs or the fetus is manipulated by the abdomen helps with the diagnosis. Speculum examination will also help to assess the length and dilatation of the cervix and to exclude cord prolapse.

INVESTIGATIONS

Diagnostic tests for rupture of membranes:

- AmniSure® (AmniSure International LLC, Boston, MA, USA): a rapid immunoassay (sensitivity of 98.9% and specificity of 100%)[28]
- Amincator® (Medical Wire & Equipment, Corsham, UK): a nitrazine test to look for pH change (sensitivity of 90%)
- ferning test: microscopic examination of the fluid which, when dried, exhibits fern-like patterns owing to the sodium chloride and protein (sensitivity of 90%, false-positive rate of 17%)
- microscopy to look for lanugo hair and fetal squames stained with Nile blue sulphate.

Tests for infection:

- full blood count to look for raised white cell count
- serum C-reactive protein: a significant elevation suggests the possibility of infection; weekly tests are not recommended
- cervical swab for bacteriological examination; weekly swabs are not performed
- low vaginal swab, sweeping across the perineum and anal canal, to identify group B streptococcus infection
- mid-stream sample of urine for microscopy and culture to exclude the possibility of urinary tract infection.

Fetal assessment:

- ultrasound examination will help identify severe oligohydramnios, confirm the fetal lie and presentation and estimate fetal weight
- cardiotocography may show evidence of possible infection if the fetal heart rate shows tachycardia with no accelerations; frequent variable decelerations may suggest cord compression owing to oligohydramnios.

MANAGEMENT

If there is no overt infection, conservative management should be considered in women who are at less than 34 weeks of gestation. Corticosteroids (betamethasone 12 mg intramuscularly in two doses, 24 hours apart) should be given to enhance fetal lung maturity. As for antibiotic cover, trials have shown that erythromycin 250 mg 6-hourly for 10 days significantly reduces chorioamnionitis and postpones preterm delivery. Penicillin can be given, but co-amoxiclav is not recommended because of the increase in necrotising enterocolitis in babies who received this drug. The role of amniocentesis is controversial, and this procedure is not recommended.

After 34 weeks of gestation, active management is advised by induction of labour with oxytocin infusion or prostaglandins. Signs of infection at any gestation are an indication for immediate delivery by induction.

The prognosis in terms of survival will depend on gestation and whether the triggering factor was infection. In general, the preterm fetus that is delivered without sepsis, hypoxia or trauma has the best prognosis.

Term prelabour rupture of membranes

Term prelabour rupture of membranes (term PROM) is defined as rupture of membranes and leakage of amniotic fluid before the onset of labour but after 37 completed weeks of gestation. Some studies have given a latent time of no painful contractions for 2 hours or 4 hours after the rupture of membranes before making a diagnosis of PROM. The incidence at term varies based on the definition used and is about 6–10%, compared with an incidence of 2–4% for PPROM.

AETIOLOGY

The factors listed below have been implicated as possible causes of term PROM:

- infection
- multiple pregnancy
- polyhydramnios
- external trauma to the abdomen
- artificial separation of membranes
- placental abruption.

CLINICAL PRESENTATION AND HISTORY

Most women will present with a history of a sudden gush of fluid which continues to drain. It might have soaked their clothes or the bed sheet and usually they can differentiate the fluid from urine.

EXAMINATION AND INVESTIGATIONS

In general terms, the clinical examination and investigations are the same as for PPROM (see page 94).

MANAGEMENT

Confirmation of the diagnosis is essential. A missed diagnosis of PROM and undue delay in initiating labour may result in chorioamnionitis, fetal infection and postpartum endomyometritis, while a wrong diagnosis of PROM and immediate induction of labour may result in failure to establish labour or poor progress in labour and an unnecessary caesarean section.

In the absence of risk factors (meconium-stained liquor or signs of infection), the woman can be given the choice of conservative management for 24–48 hours or immediate induction of labour. The various methods of induction of labour are discussed in chapter 7.

If the mother wants to have a period of conservative management, it is best to avoid a digital vaginal examination for fear of introducing infection.

Conclusion

The detailed management of labour and mode of delivery in the preterm period is not discussed in this chapter. Those with singleton cephalic presentations in labour are managed with the expectation of spontaneous vaginal delivery. There is no clear evidence of benefit of caesarean section for preterm breech presentation or multiple pregnancies, but many will choose this route, believing, without solid evidence, that caesarean delivery reduces the risk of fetal infection, hypoxia and trauma.

Advances in neonatal medicine have lowered the boundaries of viability, but caution should be exercised when dealing with infants at the borderline of viability as neonatal death and major handicap are common.

References

1. Costeloe K, Hennessy E, Gibson AT, Marlow N, Wilkinson AR. The EPICure study: outcomes to discharge from hospital for infants born at threshold of viability. *Paediatrics* 2000;106:659–71.
2. Draper ES, Manktelow B, Field DJ, James D. Prediction of survival for preterm births by weight and gestational age: retrospective population based study. *BMJ* 1999;319:1093–7.

3. Saigal S, Doyle LW. An overview of mortality and sequelae of preterm birth from infancy to adulthood. *Lancet* 2008;371:261–9.
4. Marlow N, Wolke D, Bracewell M, Samara M; EPICure Study Group. Neurologic and developmental disability at six years of age after extremely preterm birth. *N Engl J Med* 2005;352:9–19.
5. Sánchez AR, Kupp LI, Sheridan PJ, Sánchez DR. Maternal chronic infection as a risk factor in preterm low birth weight infants: the link with periodontal infection. *J Int Acad Periodontol* 2004;6:89–94.
6. Sun PM, Wilburn W, Raynor BD, Jamieson D. Sickle cell disease in pregnancy: twenty years of experience at Grady Memorial Hospital, Atlanta, Georgia. *Am J Obstet Gynecol* 2001;184:1127–30.
7. Bell SL, Norman JE. Preterm labour and delivery. In: Warren R, Arulkumaran S, editors. Best Practice in Labour and Delivery. Cambridge: Cambridge University Press; 2009. p. 216–26.
8. Ugwumadu A, Manyonda I, Reid F, Hay P. Effect of early oral clindamycin on late miscarriage and preterm delivery in asymptomatic women with abnormal vaginal flora and bacterial vaginosis: a randomised controlled trial. *Lancet* 2003;361:983–8.
9. Carey JC, Klebanoff MA, Hauth JC, Hillier SL, Thom EA, Ernest JM, et al. Metronidazole to prevent preterm delivery in pregnant women with asymptomatic bacterial vaginosis. National Institute of Child Health and Human Development Network of Maternal-Fetal Medicine Units. *N Engl J Med* 2000;342:534–40.
10. Shennan A, Crawshaw S, Briley A, Hawken J, Seed P, Jones G, et al. A randomised controlled trial of metronidazole for the prevention of preterm birth in women positive for cervicovaginal fetal fibronectin: the PREMET Study. *BJOG* 2006;113:65–74.
11. Dodd JM, Flenady V, Cincotta R, Crowther OA. Prenatal administration of progesterone for preventing preterm birth. *Cochrane Database Syst Rev* 2006;(1):CD004947.
12. Meis PJ, Klebanoff M, Thom E, Dombrowski MP, Sibai B, Moawad AH, et al.; National Institute of Child Health and Human Development Maternal-Fetal Medicine Units Network. Prevention of recurrent preterm delivery by 17 alpha-hydroxyprogesterone caproate. *N Engl J Med* 2003;348:2379–85.
13. To MS, Alfirevic Z, Heath VC, Cicero S, Cacho AM, Williamson PR, et al.; Fetal Medicine Foundation Second Trimester Screening Group. Cervical cerclage for prevention of preterm delivery in women with short cervix: randomised controlled trial. *Lancet* 2004;363:1849–53.
14. Berghella V, Rafael TJ, Szychowski JM, Rust OA, Owen J. Cerclage for short cervix on ultrasonography in women with singleton gestations and previous preterm birth: a meta-analysis. *Obstet Gynecol* 2011;117:663–71.
15. Iams JD, Goldenberg RL, Meis PJ, Mercer BM, Moawad A, Das A, et al. The length of the cervix and the risk of spontaneous preterm delivery. National Institute of Child Health and Human Development Maternal Fetal Medicine Unit Network. *N Engl J Med* 1996;334:567–72.

16. Leitich H, Kaider A. Fetal fibronectin – how useful is it in the prediction of preterm birth? *BJOG* 2003;110 Suppl 20:66–70.
17. Gyetvai K, Hannah ME, Hodnett ED, Ohlsson A. Tocolytics for preterm labor: a systematic review. *Obstet Gynecol* 1999;94:869–77.
18. Royal College of Obstetricians and Gynaecologists. *Tocolytic drugs for women in preterm labour*. Green-top Guideline. No. 1b. London: RCOG; 2011 [http://www.rcog.org.uk/womens-health/clinical-guidance/tocolytic-drugs-women-preterm-labour-green-top-1b].
19. Papatsonis D, Flenady V, Cole S, Liley H. Oxytocin receptor antagonists for inhibiting preterm labour. *Cochrane Database Syst Rev* 2005;(3):CD004452.
20. Crowther CA, Hillier JE, Doyle LW. Magnesium sulphate for preventing preterm birth in threatened preterm labour. *Cochrane Database Syst Rev* 2002;(4):CD001060.
21. Doyle LW, Crowther CA, Middleton P, Marret S, Rouse D. Magnesium sulphate for women at risk of preterm birth for neuroprotection of the fetus. *Cochrane Database Syst Rev* 2009;(1):CD004661.
22. Royal College of Obstetricians and Gynaecologists. *Antenatal corticosteroids to reduce neonatal morbidity and mortality*. Green-top Guideline No. 7. London: RCOG; 2010 [http://www.rcog.org.uk/womens-health/clinical-guidance/antenatal-corticosteroids-prevent-respiratory-distress-syndrome-gree].
23. Dessens AB, Haas HS, Koppe JG. Twenty-year follow-up of antenatal corticosteroid treatment. *Paediatrics* 2000;105:E77.
24. Kenyon SL, Taylor DJ, Mordi W; ORACLE Collaborative Group. Broad-spectrum antibiotics for spontaneous preterm labour: the ORACLE I randomised trial. ORACLE Collaborative Group. *Lancet* 2001;357:989–94.
25. Kenyon S, Pike K, Jones DR, Brocklehurst P, Marlow N, Salt A, et al. Childhood outcomes after prescription of antibiotics to pregnant women with spontaneous preterm labour: 7-year follow-up of the ORACLE II trial. *Lancet* 2008;372:1319–27.
26. Royal College of Obstetricians and Gynaecologists. *Preterm prelabour rupture of membranes*. Green-top Guideline No. 44. London: RCOG; 2010 [http://www.rcog.org.uk/womens-health/clinical-guidance/preterm-prelabour-rupture-membranes-green-top-44].
27. Carroll SG, Sebire NJ, Nicolaides KH. *Preterm prelabour amniorrhexis*. New York/London: Parthenon; 1996.
28. Cousins LM, Smok DP, Lovett SM, Poelter DM. AmniSure placental alpha microglobulin-1 rapid immunoassay versus standard diagnostic methods for detection of rupture of membranes. *Am J Perinatol* 2005;22:317–20.

9   Assisted vaginal delivery

Rates of assisted vaginal delivery with forceps and vacuum vary from country to country, within countries from hospital to hospital and within hospitals from obstetrician to obstetrician. Overall there has been a reduction in operative vaginal delivery, with some of the more difficult assisted mid-pelvis deliveries now being performed by caesarean section. The range of assisted vaginal delivery may vary between 3% and 25%, but is commonly between 5% and 12% of all deliveries. Similarly, the use of forceps and vacuum varies greatly both between and within countries. Some units will use one or the other instrument almost exclusively, but overall the use of the vacuum is increasing.[1]

CLASSIFICATION OF ASSISTED VAGINAL DELIVERY	
Outlet delivery	The fetal head is at or on the perineum and the scalp is visible without separating the labia. The head is either direct occipitoanterior or occipitoposterior or less than 45° off the anteroposterior diameter.
Low pelvis	The outlet criteria are not fulfilled but the head is at least at station +2 cm. The position may be occipitoanterior, occipitotransverse or occipitoposterior.
Mid pelvis	The fetal head is at the level of the ischial spines to station +1 cm.

Adapted from the American College of Obstetricians and Gynecologists, 2000.[2]

Indications

There are few absolute indications for assisted vaginal delivery. Most indications are relative and fall into the following broad categories:

- maternal
- fetal
- combined.

MATERNAL

● Fatigue and exhaustion leading to unproductive and non-progressive maternal effort.

● Medical condition limiting the desirability of maternal effort and the Valsalva manoeuvre, such as cardiac, cerebrovascular disease, severe pre-eclampsia, spinal cord injury.

● Maternal request.

FETAL

● Presumed fetal compromise, usually based on a suspicious or pathological fetal heart rate pattern. In these circumstances it is essential that the assisted vaginal delivery be straightforward as the combination of trauma and hypoxia is potentially damaging to the fetus.

● Acute events such as cord prolapse or placental abruption when the clinical findings are such that assisted vaginal delivery can be easily and promptly achieved.

COMBINED

In a prolonged, non-progressive second stage of labour, the decision to intervene is based on a balance of maternal and fetal reasons. Often the mother is exhausted and demoralised and her efforts are non-progressive. Prolongation may cause damage to the maternal pelvic floor.

The position of the fetal head (deflexed occipitotransverse or occipitoposterior) may present a larger diameter, contributing to the relative disproportion. Assisted vaginal delivery that corrects this deflexion will lead to a smaller diameter and easier delivery.

Prolonged arrest of the fetal head may lead to the lethal combination of fetal trauma and hypoxia. It has been suggested that when the following times are exceeded in the second stage of labour, consideration should be given to assisted delivery:[2]

● nulliparous women: 2 hours without regional anaesthesia and 3 hours with regional anaesthesia

● multiparous women: 1 hour without regional anaesthesia and 2 hours with regional anaesthesia.

However, rigid time limits should not be applied as a combination of some or all of the above maternal and fetal factors, together with balanced judgement, is needed to define the correct time for intervention.

It should also be recognised that a prolonged, non-progressive second stage carries additional morbidity for the mother and newborn.[3] The vast majority of women with a prolonged second stage and dystocia are nulliparous. A working guide to achieve a balance between excessive intervention and a laissez-faire attitude in nulliparous women is as follows.

For the first hour after full cervical dilatation, do not encourage maternal bearing-down effort. About 50% of nulliparous women will behave more like a multiparous woman and have rapid descent of the fetal head during this hour and progress to spontaneous delivery. In the remaining 50%, progress will be protracted and oxytocin augmentation should be started at the beginning of the 2nd hour.

After 1 hour of augmentation (2 hours after full dilatation), start maternal bearing-down efforts. A further hour of both oxytocin augmentation and maternal effort will complete a 3-hour second stage. At this point, one of three options should be apparent:

- Progress is such that delivery is imminent and continued maternal effort should result in spontaneous delivery.

- There is slow or arrested progress of the fetal head in the low/outlet pelvis. Discussion with the woman should guide whether she opts for assisted vaginal delivery or attempts further progress with her own effort.

- If there is arrest in the mid-pelvis, discuss the advisability of caesarean delivery.

The above approach ensures that within 3 hours, the imminent conclusion of the second stage of labour will occur and full use will have been made of oxytocin augmentation and maternal effort (Figure 9.1). This avoids the open-ended approach, which can lead to an indefinite, indecisive and interminable second stage.

Conditions to be fulfilled for assisted vaginal delivery

INDICATION AND CONSENT

In the often highly charged environment of the labour ward, it can be difficult to obtain informed consent. However, the broad options, which usually include waiting, assisted vaginal delivery or caesarean section, should be discussed with the woman. It is important to document this discussion and the indication for intervention.[4]

EFFECTIVE POWERS

One of the most important principles is that propulsion is more effective and safer than traction and extraction.[5] Thus, it is essential to use the

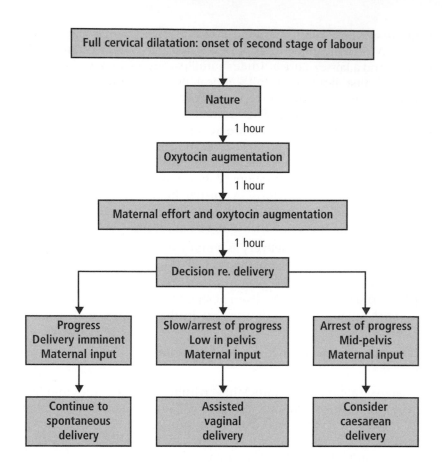

Figure 9.1 Guideline for protracted second stage of labour in nulliparous women (adapted with permission from *Munro Kerr's Operative Obstetrics*, Centenary Edition, by Thomas Baskett, Andrew Calder and Sabaratnam Arulkumaran, copyright Elsevier 2007)

uterine and maternal powers to best effect before resorting to assisted delivery. The principles of appropriate oxytocin augmentation and use of maternal effort are outlined in chapter 3.

COMBINED ABDOMINAL AND VAGINAL ASSESSMENT

A most important principle is that neither abdominal nor vaginal assessment alone provides adequate information upon which to base the decision to assist vaginal delivery. In particular, the relationship of the leading bony part of the fetal head to the ischial spines (station) can be misleading with vaginal examination alone because of the difficulties in assessing the contribution of caput and moulding to the true level of descent (Figure 9.2). In this context, the principle of assessing the fetal head in 'fifths' above the pelvic brim is important, as outlined in chapter 3, page 24. In general, if the fetal head is not palpable above the pelvic brim, the head has descended to at least spines +1 cm to +2 cm. In modern obstetrics, it is rarely indicated to assist vaginal delivery at a station higher than this, particularly if the head is arrested at this level after effective uterine and maternal effort. Thus, the abdominal palpation component of this assessment is critical and can be decisive.

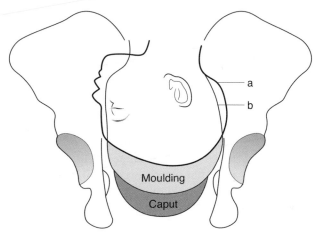

Figure 9.2 Effect of caput and moulding on apparent head level: (a) fetal head without caput and moulding; (b) fetal head after descent with caput and moulding

Other aspects of the vaginal assessment include recognising the sagittal suture and the occipital and parietal bones. The parietal bones always override the occipital bone, which is helpful in finding the posterior fontanelle. In this manner the position and the degree of flexion of the fetal head can be defined.

If the amount of caput makes this difficult, feel anteriorly for the fetal ear. Care should be taken to feel the pinna and the canal, as the ear can be folded and give a false impression of the true position of the fetus. This landmark is also useful in assessing the level of the head and the likelihood of safe assisted delivery, because the ear is just below the maximum biparietal diameter. If the ear can be easily felt during maternal bearing-down effort, significant disproportion is unlikely. The assessment of caput and moulding is outlined in chapter 3.

Synclitism is assessed by feeling the sagittal suture in its relationship to the transverse plane of the pelvic cavity. Anterior asynclitism, in which the anterior parietal bone is more easily felt and the sagittal suture further back in the transverse plane, is normal. Posterior asynclitism is a sign of disproportion.

Clinical assessment of the bony pelvis has limitations, but with experience is useful in helping to define the relationship between the fetal head and the bony pelvis. By measuring their own fingers, the obstetrician can assess the diagonal conjugate from the sacral promontory to beneath the pubic symphysis, the curve of the sacrum and the convergence of the pelvic sidewalls. The prominence of the ischial spines and sacrospinous ligaments can also be gauged. This, along with assessment of the fetal head (its position, station, degree of flexion or deflexion, asynclitism, caput, moulding and the 'feel' of how it fits in the pelvis), is an important appraisal that, if carried out at every opportunity, will allow the obstetrician to gain the experience necessary to guide safe assisted vaginal delivery.

ANALGESIA

Adequate analgesia may be provided in the form of epidural or spinal anaesthesia, pudendal block or local anaesthetic infiltration of the perineum. The amount required depends on the level of the fetal head and the need for rotation but, generally speaking, vacuum-assisted deliveries require less analgesia than forceps.

EMPTY THE BLADDER

This is best achieved by straight catheterisation just before carrying out the final combined abdominal/vaginal assessment.

TRIAL OF ASSISTED VAGINAL DELIVERY

In most cases it is clear that the head is in the low or outlet position and that assisted delivery will be accomplished with ease. However, in those cases in which the fetal head is arrested between spines +1 cm to +2 cm, it is often prudent to declare a trial of forceps or of vacuum. This entails an explanation to the woman and her partner, as well as to anaesthesia and nursing personnel, that she will be taken to the operating theatre where either assisted vaginal delivery or caesarean section can be performed. If the forceps or vacuum delivery proceeds smoothly, vaginal delivery can be safely achieved. However, if any difficulties are encountered, the obstetrician can immediately back off and proceed to caesarean section. This declaration removes any pressure from the obstetrician to persist with an attempt at vaginal delivery when difficulty is encountered. This is a very important principle and often allows safe vaginal delivery of the fetus without increasing the risk.[4,6]

GENERAL CONSIDERATIONS

When appropriate time, oxytocin augmentation and maternal effort have been used and the fetal head has arrested at spines +1 cm to +3 cm, considerable skill and circumspection is required to avoid fetal and maternal trauma. Ironically, the well-flexed, occipitoanterior fetal head that has arrested at this level may be less favourable. In contrast to the deflexed occipitotransverse or occipitoposterior positions, which when rotated to occipitoanterior will present a smaller diameter, the already well-flexed occipitoanterior head has arrested with the smallest diameter already presenting. Thus, the traction required to deliver from the apparently favourable occipitoanterior position may be greater.

CHOICE OF INSTRUMENT

There is a myth, too widely held, that vacuum-assisted delivery is associated with fewer complications and that it requires less training and skill than the use of forceps. Nothing could be further from the truth; all of the cautionary management principles outlined in this chapter apply to both instruments.

Obstetricians should be experienced in the use of both forceps and the vacuum extractor. The complications profile of each instrument is different, but one glaring difference is the failure-to-deliver rate; this is usually ≤5% with forceps but ranges from 8% to 30% with the vacuum. Failure to deliver with the vacuum is highest with fetal head malposition. In general, less analgesia is necessary for vacuum-assisted delivery than for forceps. In cases of presumed fetal compromise, assuming adequate analgesia is in place, the baby can be delivered more quickly and more assuredly with forceps than with vacuum.

Based on the clinical circumstances, and particularly on the experience of the obstetrician, the most appropriate instrument can be selected.

Forceps delivery

About 700 different types of forceps have been described, although only some two dozen are in common use. Broadly speaking, there are two types: classical forceps, used for direct traction, of which the most common are Simpson's, Neville Barnes and Haig Ferguson forceps; and specialty forceps, used for rotation and traction (Kielland's forceps) and for protection and flexion of the after-coming head of the breech (Piper's forceps).

Before embarking upon forceps delivery, ensure that the conditions appropriate for assisted vaginal delivery outlined above have been fulfilled.

CLASSICAL FORCEPS

Delivery using classical forceps is usually performed with the woman in the lithotomy position, but outlet forceps can be applied in the left lateral position if the clinical situation demands.

The pelvic findings are carefully checked and the blades of the forceps assembled and well lubricated. The handle of the left blade is held in the left hand and applied to the left side of the fetal head. The blade is held parallel to the right inguinal ligament and inserted between the fetal head and the fingers, which protect the left posterolateral vaginal wall as the blade is inserted in a circular movement to negotiate the cephalic and pelvic curves. The right blade is inserted in a similar manner (Figure 9.3).

The shanks and handles of the blades should sit horizontally: if one is at an angle and above the other blade, check for malposition or asynclitism. Slight inwards or downwards movements of the handles may be needed to 'snuggle' the blades into position. Correct application is ensured by noting that the sagittal suture is equidistant from the two blades and that there is equal space – about one fingerbreadth – between the fetal head and the 'heel' of the blade (Figure 9.4).

The occiput should be 3–4 cm above the shank. This will ensure that the line of traction is through the flexion point and that the head will present the shortest anteroposterior diameter. If the distance between the occiput and the shank is greater than 4 cm, the blades can be slightly disengaged and the handles lifted upwards and then locked when the shank is 3–4 cm below the occiput. Subsequent downward traction will flex the head and offer the most favourable anteroposterior diameter to the pelvis.

The powers of uterine contraction and maternal effort should be coordinated with steady traction downwards and backwards to negotiate the pelvic curve. Traction should not be carried out by gripping the handles but rather with the first and second fingers on the finger guards. The other hand may exert downward traction on the shanks (Pajot's manoeuvre) to ensure that traction is in the axis of the pelvic curve (Figure 9.5).

As the head descends to the pelvic floor and begins to crown, the direction of pull arches upwards to gently deliver the head and face over the perineum. Episiotomy may be required at this stage. Some will

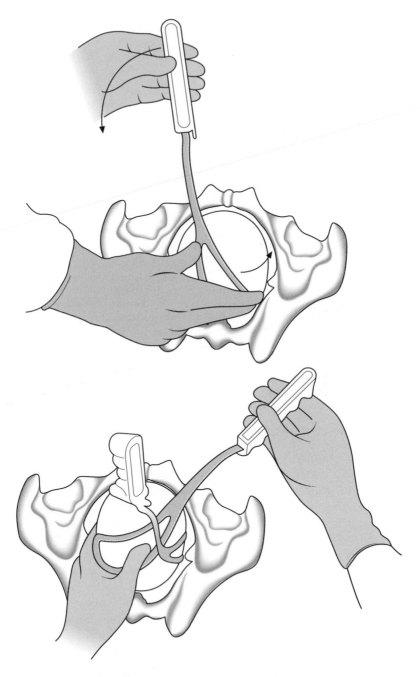

Figure 9.3 Application of classical forceps

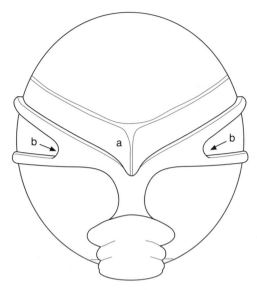

Figure 9.4 Checks for correct application of forceps in relation to the fetal head: (a) sagittal suture should be perpendicular to the shant and occiput 3–4 cm above the shank; (b) distance between heel of the blade and head is one fingerbreadth on each side

remove the handles of the forceps at this point and assist final spontaneous delivery of the head over the perineum.

ROTATIONAL FORCEPS

The most commonly used rotational forceps are those of Kielland. Considerable experience and skill are required for the safe use of this instrument.[7] Kielland's forceps are designed for rotation of the head in the occipitotransverse or occipitoposterior position. As such, there is minimal pelvic curve, thus allowing rotation without maternal trauma. Kielland's forceps also have a sliding lock to allow correction of asynclitism. By rotating the deflexed head to occipitoanterior, and in so doing flexing it as well as correcting asynclitism, the narrowest diameter of the fetal head is presented to the pelvis.

The forceps are assembled and the directional knobs on the shanks face the occiput. The two common methods of application are direct and wandering techniques (Figure 9.6). In the direct technique, the anterior blade is applied under the symphysis at an angle that facilitates and guides the blade over the curve of the fetal head. In the wandering technique, the anterior blade is applied in the traditional way along the

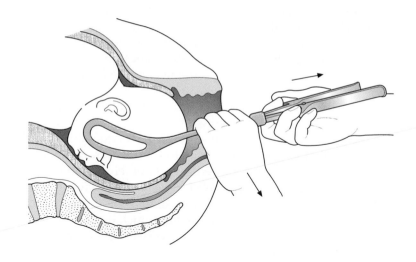

Figure 9.5 Pajot's manoeuvre

lateral vaginal wall over the sinciput or face of the fetus and then gently 'wandered' under the symphysis pubis to lie on the side of the fetal head.

In both techniques the posterior blade is applied directly. It is very important to insert the operator's hand in the posterior vagina as high as possible to protect the vaginal wall as one guides the posterior blade into position. As the tip of the blade passes the posterior aspect of the fetal head it is directed upwards, with the fingers and the handle directed downwards with the other hand to guide the blade around the fetal head. In a sense, the posterior blade is pivoted on the vaginal hand to protect the maternal tissues.

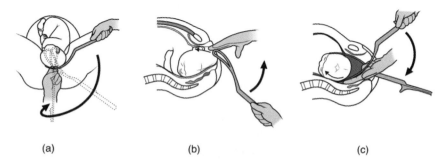

(a) (b) (c)

Figure 9.6 Application of Kielland's rotation forceps: (a) wandering application of anterior blade; (b) direct application of anterior blade; (c) application of posterior blade

The handles are locked together and the sliding lock allows correction of any asynclitism until the blades lie parallel and the handles lock easily together. As with the classical application, the relationship of the sagittal suture should be equidistant between the blades and there should be about a fingerbreadth space between the heel of the blade and the fetal head.

Rotation of the head should be carried out when the uterus is relaxed and with a very gentle, slow, progressive movement. The handles at the level of the junction with the shanks should be very gently grasped and depressed against the perineum as rotation occurs. Thus, rotation and flexion of the head should be achieved. It is extremely important to check that the head is rotating as it is possible for the blades just to move around the fixed head. Under no circumstances should force be used for this manoeuvre: either it is achieved with a light touch or it is inappropriate to continue. It is at this stage that the cervical spine and cord are vulnerable.[8]

Once rotation and flexion of the fetal head have occurred, the diameter presenting to the pelvis is reduced and can often be delivered with easy traction.

Vacuum extraction

The vacuum extractor is an alternative to forceps for assisted vaginal delivery and is gaining in popularity. It is associated with less trauma to the maternal pelvic floor and can usually be carried out with less anaesthesia. It is best not to use the vacuum at less than 34 weeks of gestation as the premature fetal head may be more vulnerable to intracranial haemorrhage.[4]

Exactly the same safeguards apply to the use of the vacuum extractor as to the forceps. Since Malmström devised the first modern vacuum extractor in the early 1950s, there have been a number of variations. Cups that have both the suction and traction points close to the middle are known as anterior cups. These are satisfactory if the head is occipito-anterior and well flexed. However, if the head is deflexed in the occipitotransverse or occipitoposterior position, the central vacuum port prevents placement of the cup laterally enough to get it over the flexion point of the fetal head.

This principle of the flexion point is central to the effective and safe application of the vacuum extractor.[9,10] In the term infant, the distance between the anterior and posterior fontanelles is approximately 9 cm. The flexion point is approximately 3 cm in front of the posterior fontanelle. Thus, when placing the centre of a 6 cm vacuum cup over the flexion point, the anterior edge of the cup will be approximately

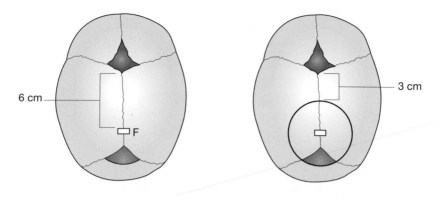

Figure 9.7 Defining the correct application of the vacuum cup over the flexion point

3 cm (about two fingerbreadths) behind the anterior fontanelle (Figure 9.7). If the cup is placed more anteriorly, it will cause deflexion and therefore a larger diameter of the fetal head will present.

If the cup is placed more to one side of the sagittal suture than the other, the application will be paramedian and present a larger diameter because of the asynclitism produced (Figure 9.8). The use of anterior cups to attempt delivery of deflexed occipitotransverse and occipito-posterior positions will often result in failure as it is impossible to guide the cup over the flexion point because of the centrally placed vacuum ports. For this reason, it is essential to have a posterior cup, as originally designed by Bird. With the suction port placed peripherally, the posterior cup allows manipulation of the cup laterally in the vagina over the flexion point of the occipitoposterior position. The principles of Bird's posterior cup have been incorporated into a new disposable rigid plastic device with an integral hand pump to create the vacuum: the Kiwi™ OmniCup (Clinical Innovations Europe, Abingdon, UK).[11,12]

Once the cup is properly applied, the vacuum is created. A finger checks around the periphery of the cup to ensure that no maternal tissue is included. There is no advantage to the slow creation of the vacuum, nor is it beneficial to reduce the vacuum between episodes of traction.

As a guiding rule, traction should be perpendicular to and within the circumference of the cup diameter to avoid cup detachment ('pop-off'). During traction with the right hand, keep the left thumb on the top of the vacuum cup and the left index finger on the scalp. The thumb provides countertraction to reduce the chance of cup release, while the index finger can gauge whether the bony part of the fetal head is descending, rather than just the scalp.

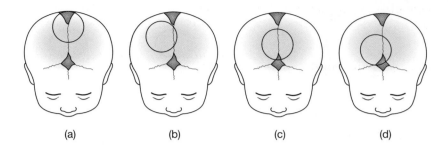

Figure 9.8 Correct and incorrect vacuum cup applications: (a) flexing median, (b) flexing paramedian, (c) deflexing median, (d) deflexing paramedian

Traction is applied during a uterine contraction, aided by maternal effort. One 'pull' equals traction during one uterine contraction. As a general rule, within three pulls it should be clear that the head is descending to the perineum. It may take several extra pulls to gently guide the head over the perineum. If the vacuum cup pops off, a very careful reappraisal should occur. One further application may be justified. Pop-offs are more common with soft cups, but this does not make them less traumatic. Soft cups are also much more likely to fail to achieve delivery than the rigid metal or plastic cups.[1,13]

Sequential instrumental delivery

The use of a second instrument to effect delivery when one instrument has failed is controversial. In clinical terms, sequential instrumental delivery usually entails the use of forceps when the vacuum has failed to deliver the baby. In large population-based studies, neonatal outcome is worse with the sequential use of instruments,[14,15] although smaller institutional reports do not show increased neonatal morbidity.[12,16] National guidelines advise caution in the use of sequential instrumental attempts at delivery.[2,4,17]

When one considers the high rate of failure to deliver with vacuum in many hospitals, the obstetrician is placed in a clinical dilemma. If, for example, the failed vacuum rate is 20%, should all those babies be delivered by caesarean section? In the majority of these cases the head has descended to station ≥3 cm and the fetal head is often on the perineum. These are the very cases in which caesarean section is most difficult, from both a maternal (extension of the uterine incision, bleeding, sepsis) and a fetal (traumatic attempts to elevate the head) point of view. The key is to distinguish between those cases in which the vacuum fails to achieve progressive descent beyond station >2 cm and those in which there has been descent to station ≥3 cm. In the former, caesarean delivery is safest, while in most of the latter cases forceps delivery can be safely undertaken.[7,12,18,19]

Complications

In general, maternal complications are higher with forceps delivery and neonatal complications more common with vacuum-assisted delivery.

MATERNAL

Vaginal lacerations and third-degree tears are more common with forceps than with vacuum, although long-term pelvic floor function is similar at 5-year follow-up.[20]

FETAL

Superficial bruising and abrasions of the face and scalp are not uncommon with forceps, but are usually trivial. Transient facial nerve palsy as a result of pressure on the seventh cranial nerve as it emerges from the stylomastoid foramen can occur. Serious cranial injuries such as depressed skull fracture and intracranial haemorrhage are rare. Cephalhaematoma is more common with vacuum than with forceps, but is self-limiting and of no long-term clinical consequence. A rare but feared complication of vacuum delivery is subgaleal haemorrhage, in which blood vessels under the aponeurosis are disrupted; bleeding into this large area may result in lethal hypovolaemia. A large review showed that the rates of subdural or cerebral haemorrhage during labour were similar in vacuum, forceps and caesarean delivery.[14] There is an increased incidence of retinal haemorrhage with vacuum extraction, but no apparent adverse long-term sequelae.

Conclusion

Both the forceps and vacuum extractor have their place in modern obstetrics and the obstetrician should be familiar with the use of both instruments. As with all surgical manoeuvres it is the judgement and skill of the person on the end of the instrument that dictates the outcome rather than the instrument itself.

For clinical audit and potential medico-legal purposes, it is essential that each assisted vaginal delivery be carefully documented immediately after delivery. This should include the indication, discussion of consent and a precise description of the station, moulding, caput, position and degree of flexion of the fetal head. A description of the procedure should follow, listing the manoeuvres, rotation, traction and level of difficulty. The number of 'pulls' should be noted. Associated episiotomy or vaginal lacerations and their repair should be described.

For some women operative vaginal delivery is seen as a defeat, and in extreme cases they will suffer a form of post-traumatic stress syndrome.[21] Some 50% of women will avoid another pregnancy following operative vaginal delivery, with fear of labour cited as the main reason.[22] Thus, in the postpartum period, a clear explanation of the events that led to the operative intervention and its implications should be given to the woman. This should include the information that, depending on the complexity of the operative delivery, there is an 80–90% chance she will deliver spontaneously in a subsequent pregnancy.[23]

References

1. Ali UA, Norwitz ER. Vacuum-assisted vaginal delivery. *Rev Obstet Gynecol* 2009;2:5–17.
2. American College of Obstetricians and Gynecologists. *Operative vaginal delivery*. ACOG Practice Bulletin No. 17. Washington DC: ACOG; 2000.
3. Allen VM, Baskett TF, O'Connell CM, McKeen D, Allen AC. Maternal and perinatal outcomes with increasing duration of the second stage of labor. *Obstet Gynecol* 2009;113:1248–58.
4. Royal College of Obstetricians and Gynaecologists. *Operative vaginal delivery*. Green-top Guideline No. 26. London: RCOG; 2011 [http://www.rcog.org. uk/womens-health/clinical-guidance/operative-vaginal-delivery-green-top-26].
5. O'Driscoll K, Meagher D, Robson M. *Active Management of Labour. Fourth edition*. London: Mosby; 2003.
6. Revah A, Ezra Y, Farine D, Ritchie K. Failed trial of vacuum or forceps – maternal and fetal outcome. *Am J Obstet Gynecol* 1997;176:200–4.
7. Baskett TF, Calder AA, Arulkumaran S. *Munro Kerr's Operative Obstetrics. Eleventh edition*. Philadelphia, USA: Saunders; 2007.
8. Menticoglou SM, Perlman M, Manning FA. High cervical spinal cord injury in neonates delivered with forceps: report of 15 cases. *Obstet Gynecol* 1995;86:589–94.
9. Bird GC. The importance of flexion in vacuum extraction delivery. *Br J Obstet Gynaecol* 1976;83:194–200.
10. Vacca A. *Handbook of Vacuum Delivery in Obstetric Practice. Third edition*. Brisbane: Vacca Research; 2009.
11. Vacca A. Operative vaginal delivery: clinical appraisal of a new vacuum extraction device. *Aust N Z J Obstet Gynaecol* 2001;41:156–60.

12. Baskett TF, Fanning CA, Young DC. A prospective observational study of 1000 vacuum assisted deliveries with the OmniCup device. *J Obstet Gynaecol Can* 2008;30:573–80.
13. O'Grady JP, Pope CS, Patel SS. Vacuum extraction in modern obstetric practice: a review and critique. *Curr Opin Obstet Gynecol* 2000;12:475–80.
14. Towner D, Castro MA, Eby-Wilkens E, Gilbert WM. Effect of mode of delivery in nulliparous women on neonatal intracranial injury. *N Engl J Med* 1999;341:1709–14.
15. Gardella C, Taylor M, Benedetti T, Hitti J, Critchlow C. The effect of sequential use of vacuum and forceps for assisted vaginal delivery on neonatal and maternal outcomes. *Am J Obstet Gynecol* 2001;185:896–902.
16. Edozien LC, Williams JL, Chatterjee IC, Hirsch PJ. Failed instrumental delivery: how safe is the use of a second instrument? *J Obstet Gynaecol* 1999;19:460–2.
17. Cargill YM, MacKinnon CJ, Arsenault MY, Bartellas E, Daniels S, Gleason T, et al.; Clinical Practice Obstetrics Committee. Guidelines for operative vaginal birth. *J Obstet Gynaecol Can* 2004;26:747–61.
18. Vacca A. Trials and tribulations of operative vaginal delivery. *BJOG* 2007;114:519–21.
19. Edozien LC. Towards safe practice in instrumental vaginal delivery. *Best Pract Res Clin Obstet Gynaecol* 2007;21:639–55.
20. Johanson RB, Heycock E, Carter J, Sultan AH, Walklate K, Jones PW. Maternal and child health after assisted vaginal delivery: five-year follow up of a randomised controlled study comparing forceps and ventouse. *Br J Obstet Gynaecol* 1999;106:544–9.
21. Murphy DJ, Pope C, Frost J, Liebling RE. Women's views on the impact of operative delivery in the second stage of labour: qualitative interview study. *BMJ* 2003;327:1132.
22. Bahl R, Strachan B, Murphy DJ. Outcome of subsequent pregnancy three years after previous operative delivery in the second stage of labour: cohort study. *BMJ* 2004;328:311.
23. Mawdsley SD, Baskett TF. Outcome of the next labour in women who had a vaginal delivery in their first pregnancy. *BJOG* 2000;107:932–4.

10 Shoulder dystocia

Shoulder dystocia occurs when there is failure of the shoulders to deliver spontaneously or with gentle downward traction on the fetal head. Shoulder dystocia is diagnosed when the head is delivered but external rotation does not occur, the head recedes with the chin firmly against the vulva and the neck is not visible or palpable. The diagnosis is, to some extent, in the eye of the beholder, which accounts for the relatively wide range of incidence: 0.2–2% of cephalic vaginal deliveries. It has been suggested that a more standard definition may be an interval between delivery of the head to completion of delivery greater than 60 seconds, or the use of ancillary manoeuvres to effect delivery of the shoulders.[1] However, even in normal deliveries without shoulder dystocia, the head may deliver with the final push of one contraction and the shoulders and rest of the infant after awaiting the next contraction. The potential for damage to the infant from asphyxia and trauma is such that shoulder dystocia has assumed considerable clinical and medico-legal significance.[2]

Mechanism

The anteroposterior diameter of the pelvic brim is narrower than the oblique and transverse diameters. The bisacromial diameter of the term fetus is larger than the biparietal diameter. Therefore, it is the flexibility of the shoulders that allows their rotation, accommodation and descent through the pelvis. In spontaneous delivery, as the head passes through the pelvic outlet the posterior fetal shoulder descends through the sciatic notch or the sacral bay, while the anterior shoulder is accommodated in the retropubic space and the obturator foramen. If the bisacromial diameter is large and the shoulders attempt to enter the pelvic brim via the narrow anteroposterior diameter, shoulder dystocia may occur. In general, the posterior shoulder will descend below the sacral promontory and it is the anterior shoulder that becomes impacted above and behind the pubic symphysis (Figure 10.1).

On rare occasions, both the anterior and the posterior shoulder may arrest above the pelvic brim, a condition known as bilateral shoulder

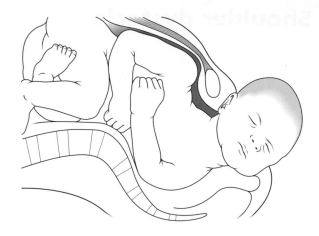

Figure 10.1 Shoulder dystocia: relationship of the anterior and posterior shoulder to the pelvic brim

dystocia. This requires considerable extension of the head and neck and is usually associated with assisted mid-pelvic delivery.

When the head delivers, the supply of oxygen to the fetus is reduced for two reasons:

- the uterus contracts down, which reduces or stops the blood flow to the intervillous space
- the fetal chest is compressed so that even though the infant's mouth and nose are delivered, effective respiratory effort is not possible.

It has been shown that after delivery of the fetal head, the progression of hypoxia is such that the umbilical artery pH falls at a rate of 0.04 units per minute.[3]

Fetal complications

ASPHYXIA

For the reasons cited above, the fetus is subjected to increasing hypoxia after delivery of the head. Provided the oxygen supply is normal until delivery of the head, there should be 4–6 minutes before the likelihood of permanent hypoxic damage. However, if there is an element of hypoxia before delivery of the head, serious asphyxia may occur in a shorter period of time. In addition, a combination of hypoxia, trauma and obstructed cerebral venous return may combine to further damage the fetal brain.

BRACHIAL PLEXUS INJURY

Brachial plexus injury is one of the most dreaded neonatal complications and has increasing medico-legal connotations. Some 5–15% of neonates born after shoulder dystocia will suffer brachial plexus palsy of the Erb–Duchenne type involving nerve roots C5 and C6. Only rarely is there injury to the whole brachial plexus leading to a flail arm. The least common injury is Klumpke's palsy, caused by damage to nerve roots C8 and T1. Fortunately, most injuries are a result of neuropraxia and recover. In those infants with brachial plexus injury, long-term disability ranges from 5% to 50%, with most series reporting permanent damage in fewer than 10% of cases.[4]

FRACTURE

The clavicle is the most likely bone to fracture and this occurs in about 15% of infants with shoulder dystocia. Fracture of the humerus does occur but much less commonly (<1%). On rare occasions, potentially disastrous fractures of the cervical spine can occur in association with twisting manoeuvres of the fetal head.

Fractures of the clavicle and humerus, when recognised and treated, heal well without long-term sequelae. While such fractures may be distressing to the accoucheur, the woman and observers, they are acknowledged complications of the condition and the manoeuvres required to treat it and do not have the same long-term implications as brachial plexus injury or severe and sustained hypoxia.

Maternal complications

GENITAL TRACT LACERATIONS

Because of the additional vaginal manoeuvres associated with shoulder dystocia, there is often extension of the episiotomy or other lacerations of the lower genital tract. Uterine rupture may occur on rare occasions in association with vigorous uterine manipulation.

POSTPARTUM HAEMORRHAGE

Postpartum haemorrhage is more common in cases of shoulder dystocia because of bleeding from lacerations and uterine atony.

Predisposing factors

ANTEPARTUM

The following factors, many of which are inter-related, increase the risk of shoulder dystocia:[5]

- Fetal macrosomia is by far the most common cause of shoulder dystocia and is often a factor in other predisposing conditions.
- Maternal diabetes: infants of women with diabetes have a greater shoulder/head circumference ratio owing to the insulin-sensitive nature of the tissues that make up shoulder girth. Such infants have a higher risk of shoulder dystocia compared with children of similar weight born to women without diabetes.
- Maternal obesity.
- Excessive maternal weight gain in pregnancy.
- Post-term pregnancy, as a result of the higher incidence of macrosomia with prolonged pregnancy. The fetal chest and shoulders will continue to grow steadily post-term, whereas the biparietal diameter growth tends to plateau, increasing the shoulder/head circumference ratio.
- Previous shoulder dystocia.

INTRAPARTUM

Although the majority of cases of shoulder dystocia show normal progression in labour leading to spontaneous or low-pelvis assisted delivery, there are certain patterns of labour that increase the likelihood of shoulder dystocia:

- protracted or arrested active phase of the late first stage of labour
- protracted or arrested descent in the second stage of labour
- assisted mid-pelvis delivery.

Prediction and prevention

Efforts have been made to find accurate predictive factors to identify a prevention strategy for shoulder dystocia and its sequelae. Unfortunately, these efforts have been unsuccessful. The main problem is that the predisposing factors are common while the condition they aim to predict, shoulder dystocia, is not. Furthermore, injury associated with shoulder dystocia is even less common.

The main risk factor is macrosomia, and the ability to predict this condition is unreliable. The hope that ultrasound would give a more precise prediction of macrosomia has not been substantiated, particularly at higher fetal weights where clinical estimates have been shown to be as accurate.[6,7] Attempts to refine ultrasound measurements using shoulder width as a predictor for shoulder dystocia have also been unsuccessful.[8]

Macrosomia is undoubtedly the most important predisposing factor to shoulder dystocia, yet the majority of cases occur in infants weighing less than 4500 g.[9] It has been suggested that if fetal weight is predicted to be over 4500 g, elective caesarean section is justified. However, the futility of such a policy was demonstrated by a decision analysis model showing that for each permanent brachial plexus injury prevented by elective caesarean section for estimated fetal weight over 4500 g, 3695 caesarean sections would have to be performed.[10] The additional cost to the health service in the USA would be US$8.7 million.

A review in 2000 of obstetric brachial palsy showed that just over 50% of all cases involved shoulder dystocia.[11] However, there is reasonable evidence from electromyographic studies that some cases of brachial plexus palsy originate in utero. There are also observational studies suggesting that the palsy may be attributable to the shoulder dystocia itself rather than the manoeuvres used to overcome it. Excessive downward traction on the head to overcome shoulder dystocia has always been implicated as the main cause of brachial plexus palsy. However, a number of studies show that in up to one-third of cases the palsy occurs in the posterior shoulder, suggesting that impaction of the posterior shoulder at the sacral promontory may be the cause.[12]

The recurrence rate of shoulder dystocia has been reviewed in seven publications, revealing a risk of recurrence ranging from 1.1% to 16.7%, with an average of about 10 %.[9,13–18] The increased risk varied from two-fold to 16-fold.

Unfortunately, therefore, we are left with predisposing factors that are common and that lack clinically applicable predictive value. Furthermore, the majority of cases of shoulder dystocia occur without identifiable risk factors. Nonetheless, awareness and appraisal of cumulative risk factors should lead to a cautious approach in selected cases. For example, a woman who has experienced a previous shoulder dystocia without injury is probably suitable for subsequent vaginal delivery, provided there are no additional risk factors and the woman is fully informed. By contrast, a woman who has experienced a previous shoulder dystocia and brachial plexus palsy, particularly if the injury was significant and sustained, is probably better delivered by elective caesarean section in a subsequent pregnancy. A woman with diabetes and a fetus whose weight is estimated to be above 4250 g is probably more safely delivered by caesarean section. Certain patterns of labour, such as a protracted late first stage of labour, slow descent in the second stage of labour and the need for assisted mid-pelvis delivery, may, in the presence of clinically diagnosed macrosomia, dictate that delivery by caesarean section would be more prudent.

Management

The classic presentation of shoulder dystocia is that the head delivers, either spontaneously or assisted, does not undergo external rotation and recoils tightly against the perineum: the so-called 'turtle sign'. If there has been no concomitant hypoxia, it is reasonable to await the next contraction and bearing-down effort for the shoulders to rotate and make their way through the pelvic brim. If this does not occur and gentle downward traction on the head fails to deliver the anterior shoulder, the presence of shoulder dystocia is clear. It is very important not to put strong downward force on the head against the unyielding anterior shoulder impacted behind the pubic symphysis; this is the most common cause of brachial plexus palsy associated with shoulder dystocia. As the problem lies at the level of the pelvic brim, traction or twisting of the fetal head and neck is illogical and potentially traumatic, and will not work. Once shoulder dystocia is diagnosed, additional personnel should be summoned to assist in providing analgesia and neonatal resuscitation and to guide the woman into the most favourable positions to assist delivery of the shoulders.

The situation should be decisively explained to the woman. Provide inhalation analgesia (if the woman is not under epidural analgesia), apply local anaesthesia to the perineum if not already in place, perform a generous episiotomy and proceed with the manoeuvres necessary to assist delivery of the shoulders, as described below.

MCROBERTS' MANOEUVRE

The McRoberts' manoeuvre is simple and the least traumatic to the fetus and mother. It will overcome the majority of mild to moderate cases of shoulder dystocia and is recommended as the first line of treatment.[19] The woman's hips are sharply flexed against her abdomen. The effect on the pelvic brim is to rotate the symphysis superiorly and straighten the lumbosacral angle. This helps to facilitate the descent of the posterior shoulder below the sacral promontory and, by flexing the fetal spine towards the anterior shoulder, may help dislodge that shoulder. It also reduces the angle of inclination of the pelvis, bringing the plane of the pelvic inlet perpendicular to the expulsive forces required for delivery (Figure 10.2). A series of engineering studies has been applied to the McRoberts' manoeuvre, showing that it does reduce the extraction

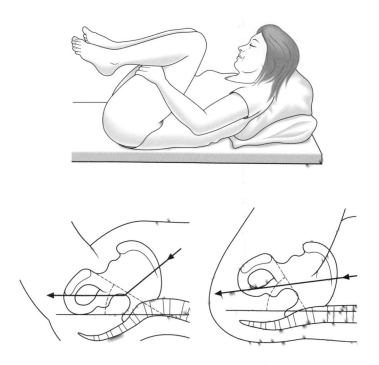

Figure 10.2 McRobert manoeuvre

forces necessary to deliver the shoulders.[20] In addition, the rate of application of force was found to be important, as fetal injury was greater when the same force was applied rapidly compared with slowly and uniformly.[21]

ROTATE THE FETAL SHOULDERS TO THE OBLIQUE DIAMETER

As the anteroposterior diameter of the pelvic brim is the narrowest, it is logical to try and rotate the shoulders to the wider oblique and transverse diameters. This should not be attempted by twisting the neck. Usually, one cannot insert fingers between the head and neck anteriorly and reach the anterior shoulder. It is best to insert the hand posteriorly in the vagina and, by pressure on the fetal axilla, push the infant's posterior shoulder off the midline to the oblique diameter. The posterior shoulder is usually accessible as it has descended below the sacral promontory.

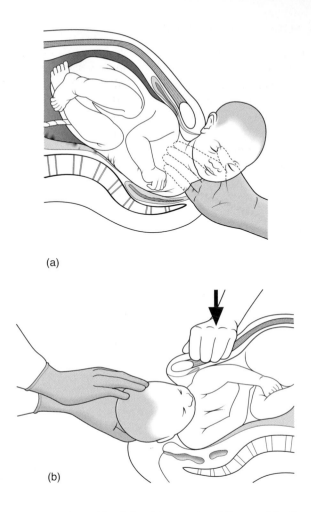

(a)

(b)

Figure 10.3 Rotation of fetal shoulders to the oblique pelvic diameter:
(a) vaginal pressure in fetal axilla; (b) suprapubic pressure

Directed suprapubic pressure may be used to assist this rotation to the oblique diameter. This pressure is best applied with the heel of the hand behind the shoulder, downwards and laterally. This pressure may be continuous or cyclical ('rocking') (Figure 10.3). Rubin showed that the adducted diameter of the shoulders is narrower than the abducted diameter, making pressure on the back of the shoulder the most logical technique.[22] There is advantage in rotating the fetal shoulders to the wider oblique diameter before or alongside all other manoeuvres.

WOODS' SCREW MANOEUVRE

In the 1940s, Woods studied the relationship between the shoulders and bony pelvis during delivery.[23] Using wooden models, he showed that the relationship between the symphysis, sacral promontory and coccyx and the fetal shoulders was similar to the threads of a screw. Woods therefore demonstrated that trying to pull or push impacted fetal shoulders through the pelvis was illogical and traumatic. However, the shoulders could be 'corkscrewed' through the pelvis by rotating the shoulders 180°. To achieve this, Woods placed two fingers on the anterior aspect of the accessible posterior shoulder in the sacral bay and exerted pressure to rotate the baby 180°. He thereby rotated the posterior shoulder, which started below the level of the pelvic brim, to the anterior position, making it accessible for delivery (Figure 10.4). The original anterior shoulder, which lay behind and above the symphysis, thus rotated below the pelvic brim to become the posterior shoulder.

In a macrosomic fetus it may not be possible to rotate the shoulders with two fingers placed in front of or behind the posterior shoulder. In these cases it is better to insert and use the whole hand, which should provide the force needed to rotate the shoulders. If this fails, the next logical step is to advance the same hand and deliver the posterior shoulder (see below).

DELIVERY OF THE POSTERIOR ARM

Delivery of the posterior arm will succeed in the vast majority of cases, except in those rare instances of bilateral shoulder dystocia where the posterior shoulder has not entered the sacral bay. Delivery of the posterior arm is achieved by passing the hand deep into the vagina along the fetal humerus to the elbow. In theory, pressure on the antecubital fossa will assist flexion of the forearm (Pinard's manoeuvre). In practice, this is not always the case, and one has to reach for the forearm, grasp the hand and wrist and deliver the posterior arm across the fetal chest (Figure 10.5). The anterior shoulder may now be accessible. If not, support the fetal head and rotate the trunk and posterior shoulder 180°, at which point the former anterior shoulder should rotate below the pelvic brim into the sacral bay and be accessible.

In cases of severe shoulder dystocia, there has been increased interest in techniques to assist delivery of the posterior arm that aim to convert the bisacromial diameter to the narrower (by up to 3 cm) axilloacromial diameter.[24] One such technique involves posterior axillary traction using the middle finger of each hand on either side into the posterior axilla of the fetus and applying traction down and out along the sacral curve.[25]

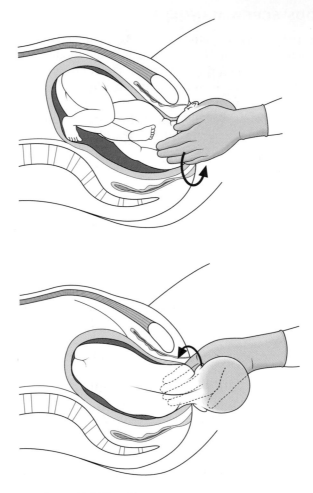

Figure 10.4 Woods' screw manoeuvre

An alternative approach is to use a plastic suction catheter as a sling around the posterior axilla for traction.[26,27]

Delivery of the posterior arm is one of the manoeuvres most likely to cause fracture of the clavicle and humerus. However, these injuries heal well without long-term disability.

ALL-FOURS MANOEUVRE

In the all-fours manoeuvre, the woman is guided to the all-fours position on her hands and knees. In this posture, gravity may help push the

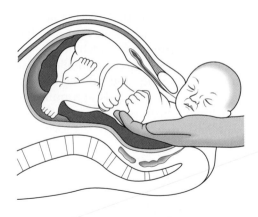

Figure 10.5 Delivery of the posterior arm

posterior shoulder forward and over the sacral promontory. In addition, the flexibility of the sacro-iliac joints may cause a 1–2 cm increase in the anteroposterior diameter of the pelvic inlet. In this position, it is the posterior shoulder that is delivered first by gentle head traction. This technique was originally observed by an American midwife working with indigenous midwives in Guatemala. There is a reported success rate of over 80% with this manoeuvre.[28] Assisting a woman with epidural analgesia into this position may require a number of personnel. Although experience with this manoeuvre is limited, the rationale and early reports suggest that it is worthwhile when standard manoeuvres have failed.

CEPHALIC REPLACEMENT (ZAVANELLI MANOEUVRE)

Cephalic replacement, or the Zavanelli manoeuvre, may have application in those rare cases of bilateral shoulder dystocia with both shoulders above the pelvic brim and inaccessible to other vaginal manoeuvres. The mechanism of delivery is reversed by grasping the fetal head in the hand, flexing it and returning it to the vagina. In many cases, this is apparently accomplished with greater ease than one would expect. On other occasions, uterine relaxation may have to be provided using nitro-glycerine or terbutaline. The fetal heart is monitored while preparations are made to deliver the infant by caesarean section. Cases have been recorded where more than 1 hour has elapsed between replacement of the head, followed by normal fetal heart rate recording and safe delivery by caesarean section. The success rate reported is in excess of 90%, but there is significant associated maternal morbidity, with ruptured uterus in some 5% and blood transfusion in 10%. Perinatal death and morbidity associated with asphyxia and brachial plexus palsy have occurred in a significant minority of infants, much of which may be associated with the delay and manoeuvres that preceded the cephalic replacement.[29]

Although cephalic replacement and subsequent caesarean section seems a radical procedure, experience is accumulating to suggest that this approach is worthwhile in those rare cases of shoulder dystocia in which the more standard manoeuvres to achieve vaginal delivery are unsuccessful.

ABDOMINAL RESCUE

Rare cases of so-called abdominal rescue have been described following failed cephalic replacement. If the head cannot be replaced high enough in the vagina to allow its delivery by caesarean section, a lower-segment uterine incision is made. By direct manipulation, the anterior shoulder 'pops up', allowing descent of the posterior shoulder and direct rotation of the anterior shoulder to the oblique diameter so that the posterior shoulder becomes accessible for manoeuvres to allow vaginal delivery of the infant.[30]

SYMPHYSIOTOMY

Although symphysiotomy has been suggested for cases of shoulder dystocia that are refractory to other manoeuvres, there are no published series of its successful use for this purpose. One recent report of three cases from the USA showed poor infant outcome and significant maternal morbidity.[31] Symphysiotomy continues to have a place in developing countries for carefully selected cases of cephalopelvic disproportion. Those experienced with the procedure can perform it under local anaesthesia in less than 5 minutes. While symphysiotomy has theoretical potential for the management of rare cases of shoulder dystocia, it is unlikely to gain acceptance in developed countries where experience with the procedure is limited or non-existent.

CLEIDOTOMY

Cleidotomy is often quoted as an alternative procedure in cases of shoulder dystocia. However, the deliberate fracture or cutting of the clavicle is not easy to achieve in the term fetus. Furthermore, there is the potential for trauma to the underlying subclavian vessels and brachial plexus. Thus, this procedure is really considered only for the fetus that is dead or has a lethal anomaly.

FUNDAL PRESSURE

The use of fundal pressure in shoulder dystocia is controversial and is often condemned in the medico-legal arena. Used in isolation, fundal pressure has no role and may serve only to compound the impaction of the anterior shoulder behind the symphysis. When maternal efforts are inadequate, particularly with regional anaesthesia, fundal pressure has been used to assist delivery. This is highly controversial and is not recommended.[33]

There are few more composure-testing moments in the life of the accoucheur than those spent dealing with shoulder dystocia. An understanding of the mechanisms involved and the manoeuvres necessary to overcome the dystocia is essential for all labour ward personnel. A clear plan and sequence of manoeuvres should be laid out and practised by all involved with the care of women in labour. There is some evidence that drills and simulation training may be of benefit.[32]

After a case of shoulder dystocia it is important, for clinical audit and medico-legal purposes, that the accoucheur clearly writes in the chart the type, timing and sequence of manoeuvres used.[33] Events should also be reviewed with the mother and well-coordinated efforts made for support and follow-up if the infant has been injured.

References

1. Spong CY, Beall M, Rodrigues D, Ross MG. An objective definition of shoulder dystocia: prolonged head-to-body delivery intervals and/or the use of ancillary obstetric maneuvers. *Obstet Gynecol* 1995;86:433–6.
2. Leigh TH, James CE. Medico-legal commentary: shoulder dystocia. *Br J Obstet Gynaecol* 1998;105:815–17.
3. Wood C, Ng KH, Houndslow D, Benning H. Time – an important variable in normal delivery. *J Obstet Gynaecol Br Commonw* 1973;80:295–300.
4. Pondaag W, Malessy MJ, van Dijk JG, Thomeer RT. Natural history of obstetric brachial plexus palsy: a systematic review. *Develop Med Child Neurol* 2004;46:138–44.
5. Baskett TF. Shoulder dystocia. *Best Pract Res Clin Obstet Gynaecol* 2002;16:57–68.
6. Chauhan SP, Hendrix NW, Magann EF, Morrison JC, Kenney SP, Devoe LD. Limitations of clinical and sonographic estimates of birth weight: experience with 1034 parturients. *Obstet Gynecol* 1998;91:72–7.
7. Sherman DJ, Arieli S, Tovbin J, Siegel G, Caspi E, Bukovsky I. A comparison of clinical and ultrasonic estimation of fetal weight. *Obstet Gynecol* 1998;91:212–7.
8. Verspyck E, Goffinet F, Hellot MF, Milliez J, Marpau L. Newborn shoulder width: a prospective study of 2222 consecutive measurements. *Br J Obstet Gynaecol* 1999;106:589–93.

9. Baskett TF, Allen AC. Perinatal implications of shoulder dystocia. *Obstet Gynecol* 1995;86:14–7.
10. Rouse DJ, Owen J, Goldenberg RL, Cliver SP. The effectiveness and costs of elective cesarean delivery for fetal macrosomia diagnosed by ultrasound. *JAMA* 1996;276;1480–6.
11. Pollack RN, Buchman AS, Yaffe H, Divon MY. Obstetrical brachial palsy: pathogenesis, risk factors, and prevention. *Clin Obstet Gynecol* 2000;43:236–46.
12. Walle T, Hartikainen-Sorri AL. Obstetric shoulder injury. Associated risk factors, prediction, and prognosis. *Acta Obstet Gynecol Scand* 1993;72:450–4.
13. Smith RB, Lance C, Pearson JF. Shoulder dystocia: what happens at the next delivery? *Br J Obstet Gynaecol* 1994;101:713–5.
14. Lewis DF, Raymond RC, Perkins MB, Brooks GG, Heymann AR. Recurrence rate of shoulder dystocia. *Am J Obstet Gynecol* 1995;172:1369–71.
15. Flannelly G, Simm A. A study of delivery following shoulder dystocia. Proceedings of the British Congress of Obstetrics and Gynaecology. 4–7 July 1995. Dublin, Ireland. Abstract 516.
16. Olugbile A, Mascarenhas L. Review of shoulder dystocia at the Birmingham Women's Hospital. *J Obstet Gynaecol* 2000;20:267–70.
17. Ginsberg NA, Moisidis C. How to predict recurrent shoulder dystocia. *Am J Obstet Gynecol* 2001;184:1427–9; discussion 1429–30.
18. Moore HM, Reed SD, Batra M, Schiff MA. Risk factors for recurrent shoulder dystocia: Washington state, 1987–2004. *Am J Obstet Gynecol* 2008;198:e16–24.
19. Gonik B, Stringer CA, Held B. An alternate maneuver for management of shoulder dystocia. *Am J Obstet Gynecol* 1983;145:882–4.
20. Gonik B, Allen R, Sorab J. Objective evaluation of the shoulder dystocia phenomenon: effect of maternal pelvic orientation on force reduction. *Obstet Gynecol* 1989;74:44–8.
21. Allen RH, Bankoski BR, Butzin CA, Nagey DA. Comparing clinician-applied loads for routine, difficult, and shoulder dystocia deliveries. *Am J Obstet Gynecol* 1994;171:1621–7.
22. Rubin A. Management of shoulder dystocia. *JAMA* 1964;189:835–7.
23. Woods CE. A principle of physics as applicable to shoulder delivery. *Am J Obstet Gynecol* 1943;45:796–805.
24. Kung J, Swan AV, Arulkumaran S. Delivery of the posterior arm reduces shoulder dystocia dimensions in shoulder dystocia. *Int J Gynaecol Obstet* 2006;93:233–7.
25. Menticoglou SM. A modified technique to deliver the posterior arm in severe shoulder dystocia. *Obstet Gynecol* 2006;108:755–7.
26. Cluver CA, Hofmeyr GJ. Posterior axilla sling traction: a technique for intractable shoulder dystocia. *Obstet Gynecol* 2009;113:486–8.
27. Gherman R. Posterior axillary sling traction: another empiric technique for shoulder dystocia alleviation? *Obstet Gynecol* 2009;113:478–9.
28. Bruner JP, Drummond SB, Meenan AL, Gaskin IM. All-fours maneuver for reducing shoulder dystocia during labor. *J Reprod Med* 1998;43:439–43.

29. Sandberg EC. The Zavanelli maneuver: 12 years of recorded experience. *Obstet Gynecol* 1999;93:312–7.
30. O'Leary JA, Cuva A. Abdominal rescue after failed cephalic replacement. *Obstet Gynecol* 1992;80:514–6.
31. Goodwin TM, Banks E, Miller LK, Phalen JP. Catastrophic shoulder dystocia and emergency symphysiotomy. *Am J Obstet Gynecol* 1997;177:463–4.
32. Crofts JF, Bartlett C, Ellis D, Hunt LP, Fox R, Draycott TJ. Management of shoulder dystocia: skill retention 6 and 12 months after training. *Obstet Gynecol* 2007;110:1069–74.
33. Royal College of Obstetricians and Gynaecologists. *Shoulder dystocia.* Green-top Guideline No. 42. London: RCOG; 2005 [http://www.rcog.org.uk/womens-health/clinical-guidance/shoulder-dystocia-green-top-42].

11 Breech vaginal delivery

The fetus presents by the breech in 3–4% of all deliveries, making it the most common malpresentation. Since the last decade of the 20th century, debate has continued as to whether the breech fetus is more safely delivered by caesarean section or by assisted vaginal delivery in selected cases.[1–3] During this time most obstetricians in developed countries 'voted with their scalpels', such that there was a steady increase in the proportion of breeches delivered by caesarean section. For many the debate was answered in favour of caesarean delivery with the publication in 2000 of the Term Breech Trial,[4] a Canadian-organised international multicentre randomised trial. Indeed, elective caesarean delivery of the breech fetus was widely adopted and in at least one national survey recorded an improvement in neonatal outcome.[5] Thus, where facilities existed, the standard of care became elective caesarean delivery for the fetus in breech presentation at term. Although the Term Breech Trial showed a significant improvement in neonatal mortality and morbidity with elective caesarean delivery,[4] the infant outcome at 2 years of age was similar in both groups.[6] In recent years there have been publications advocating selective vaginal delivery of the term breech, supported in some cases by institutional data.[7–10] Some national guidelines have been modified to support those obstetricians willing to offer selective vaginal delivery, although the vast majority of cases are still delivered by caesarean section.[11–13]

Although the Term Breech Trial applied only to the term breech, most obstetricians also deliver the preterm breech fetus by caesarean section, without objective evidence that it is safer for the neonate.

Despite the intention to deliver all viable breech presentations by caesarean section, there will be occasions when vaginal delivery is unavoidable. Furthermore, the principles of atraumatic assisted vaginal breech delivery also apply to delivery of the breech through a uterine incision. It is for these reasons that we have included this chapter on breech vaginal delivery.

The need for vaginal breech delivery may arise under the following circumstances:

- labour and delivery occur in a site where immediate caesarean section is not available

- the woman arrives at hospital in advanced labour with the breech already on the perineum

- incorrect diagnosis of the presenting part, such that a frank breech is mistaken for a cephalic presentation until late in the second stage of labour

- the woman may decide, even after being fully informed of the risks, that she wishes to proceed with vaginal delivery.

One of the problems with an almost universal policy of breech delivery by caesarean section is that it becomes a self-fulfilling prophecy that those in training will have inadequate exposure to assisted breech vaginal delivery.[14] However, theoretical and practical training can be achieved using manikins and, as mentioned above, most of the manoeuvres required for safe delivery of the breech through the uterine incision are similar to those required for assisted vaginal delivery.[15,16] A disciplined and systematic approach to each case delivered by caesarean section can therefore help provide the skills for those rare occasions when one is called upon to conduct a vaginal breech delivery.

In essence, the risks to the fetus in breech presentation are as follows:

- as a group, fetuses in breech presentation have a higher risk of intrinsic abnormalities than those with cephalic presentation; these abnormalities may range from obvious anomalies to more subtle neurological abnormalities, which may account for the overall worse outcome for breech infants irrespective of the method of delivery[3]

- asphyxia during labour is more common as a result of cord entanglement and/or prolapse

- intra-abdominal trauma owing to excessive manipulation with the operator's hands encroaching on the fetal abdomen

- trauma to the fetal limbs, particularly in association with extended or nuchal arms

- cervical spine injuries from excessive traction or torsion

- brachial plexus injuries from traction on the fetal body during attempts to deliver the head

- sudden decompression of the fetal head at the point of delivery causing tentorial tears and intracranial haemorrhage.

Unfavourable factors that may preclude safe vaginal delivery of the fetus in breech presentation include:[11]

- footling breech (Figure 11.1)

- fetal growth restriction

- extremes of fetal weight: less than 2000 g or over 3800 g

- hyperextended fetal neck in labour (best checked with ultrasound)
- clinically inadequate pelvis
- lack of a clinician trained in vaginal breech delivery.

Management of breech delivery

The guiding principle is to allow the infant to deliver spontaneously with the minimum of intervention. However, a few specific points of assistance – particularly protective delivery of the head – are required to avoid injury.

FIRST STAGE OF LABOUR

If the first stage of labour is uneventful and progressive, a safe vaginal delivery is likely. Both the frank and complete types of breech are reasonable dilators of the cervix.

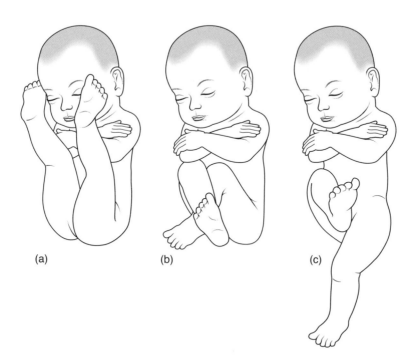

(a)   (b)   (c)

Figure 11.1 Types of breech presentation: (a) frank; (b) complete; (c) footling

Umbilical cord compression owing to entanglement or prolapse is more common with breech presentations and should be routinely excluded by pelvic examination after rupture of the membranes or if there is abnormality of the fetal heart rate.

One of the great potential hazards is caused by the breech and trunk of the fetus being smaller in diameter than the after-coming head. This is even more exaggerated in the premature infant. Thus, it is possible for the breech and legs to appear at the introitus through an incompletely dilated cervix. If delivery is attempted, the dreaded complication of entrapment of the fetal head by an incompletely dilated cervix is realised. It is therefore essential in all cases to ensure that the cervix is fully dilated and retracted before proceeding with delivery.

ANAESTHESIA

In many instances, provided it gives the woman adequate analgesia, the combination of narcotic, inhalation and pudendal block analgesia allows the most natural progression of the first and second stages of labour. However, there is much to be gained with epidural analgesia, particularly in preventing premature maternal bearing-down effort in the late first and early second stages of labour before the cervix has fully dilated and completely retracted into the lower uterine segment. On the other hand, one wants full maternal effort during the second stage, so a selective type of epidural that allows retention of motor function is the ideal. An anaesthetist should be present at all breech deliveries for the rare case when rapid general anaesthesia or uterine relaxation is required.

DELIVERY OF THE BREECH AND LEGS

The key point is 'hands off the breech'. In general, manoeuvres involving rotation and flexion of the limbs and trunk are helpful while those involving traction are not. The breech should be allowed to descend to the perineum with maternal effort alone. At this point the woman can be placed in the lithotomy position and, if appropriate, a pudendal block performed along with local anaesthetic infiltration of the perineum.

As the breech meets the opposition of the perineum, the anterior buttock 'climbs up' the fourchette. Once the anterior buttock ascends to the point where the fetal anus is visible over the fourchette, which is usually heralded by a bead of meconium, the point has been reached when further spontaneous progression will occur only when the obstruction of the perineum has been removed by a generous medio-lateral episiotomy. In a footling breech, the point at which episiotomy should be performed is when the buttocks reach the perineum. In a multiparous woman with a lax perineum, an episiotomy may not be necessary.

Wait until the beginning of a contraction before performing the episiotomy. This will allow maternal effort during one entire uterine contraction to help deliver the buttocks and legs. Here again it is appropriate to keep your hands off the breech and allow spontaneous progression. Only if it is a frank breech with extended legs will assistance be necessary in the form of two fingers placed behind the fetal thigh to flex the hip and knee and allow delivery of the leg. This is performed for each leg in turn. The remainder of the fetal abdomen and lower trunk will then follow by maternal effort alone.

Check that the umbilical cord is not under undue tension and, if it is, gently hook down a loop of cord.

The fetal back will usually remain anterolateral during this time. If the back shows any tendency to rotate posteriorly, it should be gently guided to the anterior position. It is very important not to put traction on the fetus at this point, as this will serve only to extend the fetal arms and head. This requires discipline, as one instinctively wants to aid the process of delivery. So, other than the few manoeuvres required above, continue to keep your hands off the breech.

DELIVERY OF THE SHOULDERS AND ARMS

With maternal effort alone, the remainder of the trunk should be expelled and the lower border of one scapula will become visible under the pubic arch. The fetal head is now entering the pelvic brim and the umbilical cord will be partially or completely occluded. One should note the time on the clock and plan to have the delivery complete within the next 2–3 minutes. This is when fine judgement is required to run the gauntlet between excessive haste and potentially traumatic delivery and waiting too long so that hypoxia will supervene.

Once the scapula is visible, the arms will probably be flexed in front of the fetus. Delivery of the arms, if not spontaneous, can easily be achieved by passing the index and middle fingers over the shoulder and then splinting and sweeping the humerus down across the chest. The fetal back is rotated 90° to bring the other scapula into view and the procedure repeated on the other arm.

For rotation of the fetal back or other manoeuvres required to deliver extended arms (see below), appropriate placement of the operator's hands is important. The instinct is to grasp the infant around the hips and abdomen. This is potentially traumatic to the intra-abdominal contents. The hands must be placed lower than this, around the thighs and hips of the fetus, so that the thumbs are on the sacrum and the upper fingers around the iliac crest. A small sterile towel will help maintain the grip during this manoeuvre.

EXTENDED ARMS

When extended arms occur it is usually because inappropriate traction has been placed on the fetus before this point. Løvset's manoeuvre is a very effective way of dealing with this complication. This manoeuvre is based on the principle that the posterior fetal shoulder enters the maternal pelvic cavity before the anterior shoulder.

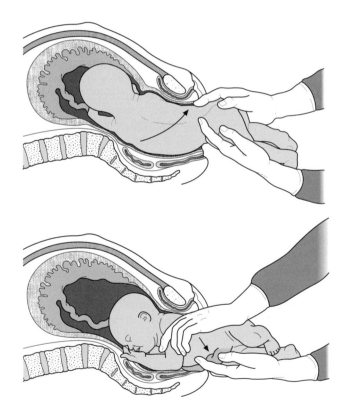

Figure 11.2 Løvset's manoeuvre
Lateral flexion is exaggerated to facilitate descent of the posterior shoulder beneath the sacral promontory. With the back uppermost, the body is rotated 180°. The posterior shoulder has now been rotated anteriorly beneath the symphysis and can be hooked down. The body is then rotated 180° and the other arm delivered in the same way.

In the manner mentioned above, the fetal thighs and hips are grasped and the body lifted anteriorly to cause lateral flexion and promote descent of the posterior shoulder below the sacral promontory. The fetal back is kept uppermost as the body is rotated 180° so that the posterior shoulder (below the pelvic brim) is now rotated to become the anterior shoulder. As such, the shoulder is now below the symphysis and the humerus can be hooked down with ease. The body is then rotated back through 180°, which brings the other shoulder below the symphysis and allows delivery of that arm (Figure 11.2).

NUCHAL ARM

In the situation with nuchal arm, the shoulder is extended and the elbow flexed so that the forearm is trapped behind the occiput. This may occur because of inappropriate traction and rotational maneouvres at an earlier stage in the delivery. To overcome this problem, the fetal trunk is rotated in the direction of the fetal hand (Figure 11.3). The occiput thus rotates past the arm and, with further rotation, flexion of the shoulder should occur and allow delivery of the arm.

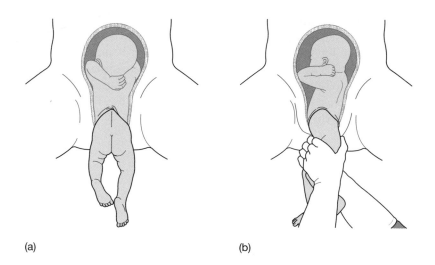

(a)   (b)

Figure 11.3 Nuchal arm
The body is rotated 90°, freeing the forearm from behind the occiput. The friction of rotation promotes flexion of the shoulder, making it accessible for delivery.

DELIVERY OF THE HEAD

After delivery of the arms, the baby is suspended vertically with partial support from the operator's hands. Mild suprapubic pressure from an assistant may help descent and flexion of the fetal head. The baby should not be allowed to hang entirely by its own weight as this may, paradoxically, promote extension of the head.

Once the hairline on the fetal neck is visible beneath the pubic arch, the head is ready for assisted delivery. Assistance at this stage is necessary to avoid sudden decompression of the perineum on the fetal head at the point of delivery. This 'champagne cork' delivery can lead to tentorial tears and intracranial haemorrhage. For this reason the head must be controlled at delivery in all cases. There are two main techniques to achieve this: forceps to the after-coming head and the Mauriceau–Smellie–Veit manoeuvre.

Forceps to the after-coming head

Forceps to the after-coming head is usually the best method and provides the most efficient protection and controlled delivery of the fetal head. An additional asset of forceps is that they encourage flexion of the head and are the safest way to apply the mild traction that may be necessary to complete delivery.

While an assistant holds the fetal body just above the horizontal plane, the forceps are applied below the body at the 4 and 8 o'clock positions along the sides of the fetal head (Figure 11.4). Most long-handled forceps can be used, but Piper's forceps were specially developed for this purpose as they have a long shank. At this stage it is important not to allow the fetal body to be raised much above the horizontal, as this risks hyperextension of and trauma to the fetal cervical spine. As the head is delivering, and once the fetal chin and mouth are visible, the forceps and the body of the fetus are raised in unison to complete delivery.

Mauriceau–Smellie–Veit manoeuvre

The Mauriceau–Smellie–Veit manoeuvre does not provide quite the same degree of protection and control as forceps. However, it can be very useful when events happen so rapidly that application of forceps is not feasible.

The operator's forearm is placed under the fetal body so that it lies astride the forearm. The forefinger and middle fingers are placed on the maxilla beside the nose to promote flexion of the fetal head. The other hand is placed on the fetal back, the middle finger pushing upwards on the occiput to enhance flexion of the head with the other fingers resting on the fetal shoulders (Figure 11.5). In this manner the cervical spine is

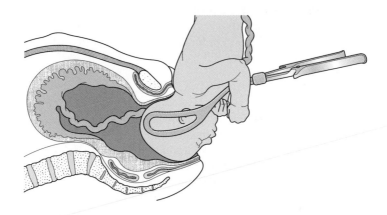

Figure 11.4 Breech delivery: forceps to the after-coming head

splinted and protected. Gentle traction in a downward and backward direction may be necessary until delivery of the fetal chin is followed by upward guidance of the face and forehead over the perineum. In many cases, it is more a matter of trying to hold back and control delivery of the head to avoid sudden decompression. Indeed, it is inappropriate to use the Mauriceau–Smellie–Veit manoeuvre to apply traction as this risks trauma to the brachial plexus and cervical spine. If more than very mild traction is needed, the traction should be applied with forceps, as described above.

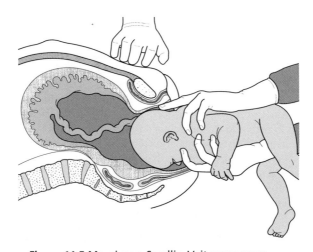

Figure 11.5 Mauriceau–Smellie–Veit manoeuvre

The fact that the vast majority of breech fetuses are delivered by caesarean section means that it is important to organise clinical services to provide skilled external cephalic version to reduce the incidence of breech presentation at term.[17]

References

1. Cheng M, Hannah M. Breech delivery at term: a critical review of the literature. *Obstet Gynecol* 1993;82:605–18.
2. Gifford DS, Morton SC, Fiske M, Kahn K. A meta-analysis of infant outcomes after breech delivery. *Obstet Gynecol* 1995;85:1047–54.
3. Danielian PJ, Wang J, Hall MH. Long-term outcome by method of delivery of fetuses in breech presentation at term: population based follow up. *BMJ* 1996;312:1451–3.
4. Hannah ME, Hannah WJ, Hewson SA, Hodnett ED, Saigal S, Willan AR. Planned caesarean section versus planned vaginal birth for breech presentation at term: a randomised multicentre trial. Term Breech Trial Collaborative Group. *Lancet* 2000;356:1375–83.
5. Rietberg CC, Elferink-Stinkens PM, Visser GH. The effect of the Term Breech Trial on medical intervention behaviour and neonatal outcome in The Netherlands: an analysis of 35,453 term breech infants. *BJOG* 2005;112:205–9.
6. Whyte H, Hannah ME, Saigal S, Hannah WJ, Hewson S, Amankwah K, et al.; Term Breech Trial Collaborative Group. Outcomes of children at 2 years after planned cesarean birth versus planned vaginal birth for breech presentation at term: the International Randomized Term Breech Trial. *Am J Obstet Gynecol* 2004;191:864–71.
7. Van Roosmalen J, Rosendaal F. There is still room for disagreement about vaginal delivery of breech infants at term. *BJOG* 2002;109:967–9.
8. Alarab M, Regan C, O'Connell MP, Keane DP, O'Herlihy C, Foley ME. Singleton vaginal breech delivery at term: still a safe option. *Obstet Gynecol* 2004;103:407–12.
9. Turner MJ. The Term Breech Trial: are the clinical guidelines justified by the evidence? *J Obstet Gynaecol* 2006;26:491–4.
10. Goffinet F, Carayol M, Foidart JM, Alexander S, Uzan S, Subtil D, et al.; PREMODA Study Group. Is planned vaginal delivery for breech presentation at term still an option? Results of an observational prospective survey in France and Belgium. *Am J Obstet Gynecol* 2006;194:1002–11.
11. Royal College of Obstetricians and Gynaecologists. *The management of breech presentation*. Green-top Guideline No. 20b. London: RCOG; 2006 [http://www.rcog.org.uk/womens-health/clinical-guidance/management-breech-presentation-green-top-20b].
12. ACOG Committee on Obstetric Practice. ACOG Committee Opinion No. 340. Mode of term singleton breech delivery. *Obstet Gynecol* 2006;108:235–7.

13. Kotaska A, Menticoglou S, Gagnon R, Farine D, Basso M, Bos H, et al.; Maternal Fetal Medicine Committee; Society of Obstetricians and Gynaecologists of Canada. Vaginal delivery of breech presentation. *J Obstet Gynecol Can* 2009;31:557–66, 567–78.

14. Chinnock M, Robson S. Obstetric trainees' experience in vaginal breech delivery: implications for future practice. *Obstet Gynecol* 2007;110:900–3.

15. Baskett TF. Trends in operative obstetrical delivery: implications for specialist training. *Ann R Coll Physicians Surg Can* 1988;1:1119–21.

16. Queenan JT. Teaching infrequently used skills; vaginal breech delivery. *Obstet Gynecol* 2004;103:405–6.

17. Royal College of Obstetricians and Gynaecologists. *External cephalic version and reducing the incidence of breech presentation.* Green-top Guideline No. 20a. London: RCOG; 2006 [http://www.rcog.org.uk/womens-health/clinical-guidance/external-cephalic-version-and-reducing-incidence-breech-presentation].

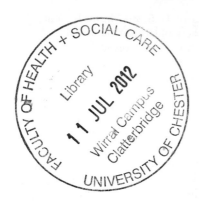

12 Twin and triplet delivery

Since the mid-1990s, as a result of assisted reproductive technology, the incidence of twin pregnancy has doubled and the number of triplets has increased ten-fold.[1] Compared with singleton pregnancies, the perinatal morbidity and mortality of twins is increased five- to ten-fold and to a much greater degree for triplets and higher-order multiple births. Overall, multiple pregnancies account for about 3% of all births but contribute approximately 25% of early preterm births (less than 32 weeks of gestation), low-birthweight infants (under 2500 g), and very low-birthweight infants (under 1500 g).[2] Compared with singletons, the incidence of cerebral palsy is increased eight-fold in twins and about 40-fold with triplets.[3,4] The main determinants of this increase in morbidity and mortality are prematurity, growth restriction, anomalies and twin-to-twin transfusion.[5] Asphyxia and trauma during delivery make a smaller contribution to morbidity and mortality but can be all the more tragic when the safe conclusion of a high-risk pregnancy is at hand. It is therefore understandable that in many developed countries the caesarean section rate for twins has roughly doubled, from 25% to 50%, since the mid-1990s, although there is no proof that abdominal delivery is safer for the infants. An international randomised trial is under way to determine the safest mode of delivery.

However, it is clear that, irrespective of the mode of delivery, twins should be delivered in hospitals with adequate anaesthetic, obstetric and neonatal personnel and facilities.

Obstetric factors

At the time of delivery, the most common presentations in twin pregnancies are (twin A/twin B):

- vertex/vertex
- vertex/breech
- breech/vertex
- breech/breech.

his covers more than 90% of the combinations, with the remainder
volving transverse lie of one or both fetuses. In practical terms, the
most common combinations are:

- vertex/vertex: 40%
- vertex/non-vertex: 35–40%
- non-vertex/other: 20–25%.

Thus, in 75–80% of cases the first twin is in cephalic presentation and
this will be the dominant factor in the decision to allow labour and
vaginal delivery. There are those who feel that if the second twin is in
a non-vertex position at the start of labour, caesarean section is
justified. However, in about 20% of cases the position of the second
twin will change after delivery of the first, and may go from an
unfavourable to a favourable position or, alternatively, from a
favourable to an unfavourable lie. In addition, the option is available
for version of the second twin should it be in an unfavourable presentation or, in extreme cases, delivery of the second twin by caesarean
section. Thus, the lie or presentation of the second twin at the start of
labour should not influence the decision to allow labour and vaginal
delivery.

Individual factors, however, will influence the decision for or against
labour and vaginal delivery. This will include the availability of appropriate facilities and personnel. Clinical factors to be evaluated include:

- extremes of estimated fetal weight (less than 1500 g or more than
  3500 g)
- weight discrepancy between twins A and B (particularly if twin B is
  larger than twin A)
- potential fetal compromise from growth restriction or twin-to-twin
  transfusion.

Maternal considerations will include age, parity, history of infertility and
previous obstetric factors such as caesarean section. Monochorionic,
monoamniotic placentation accounts for only 1% of all twins, but the
risk of cord and fetal entanglement is such that all such cases should be
delivered by elective caesarean section.[6]

The second twin faces potential increased risks during labour. After the
first twin has been delivered, the reduction in uterine size or partial
placental separation may reduce blood flow to the intervillous space,
creating hypoxia. There is also a greater risk of trauma to the second
twin owing to the intrauterine manipulations required for malpresentation.

Anaesthetic factors

There is much in favour of epidural analgesia for twin delivery. If epidural is unavailable, pudendal block and local infiltration of the perineum performed just before delivery of the first twin should allow most of the vaginal manipulations required to deliver the second twin.

Epidural is the ideal as it will allow both vaginal and intrauterine manipulations and cover the unlikely need to deliver the second twin by caesarean section. The limitation of epidural anaesthesia is the fact that it does not cause uterine relaxation. This is of critical importance if delivery of the second twin by internal version and breech extraction is undertaken. In these cases, the choice is either to superimpose general anaesthesia on top of the epidural or to provide short-term uterine relaxation with intravenous glyceryl trinitrate. The latter is more acceptable. This is one of a number of uses for emergency short-term uterine relaxation with glyceryl trinitrate; the details of its administration are covered in chapter 23 (page 246). Obstetric anaesthetists and obstetricians must be aware of the need for complete uterine relaxation to safely carry out internal version and breech extraction for the second twin.

Management of labour

FIRST STAGE OF LABOUR

The first stage of labour is managed as for a singleton fetus. If the first twin is other than a vertex presentation, it will probably be delivered by elective caesarean section. If possible, both twins should receive fetal heart rate monitoring during labour. Oxytocin induction and/or augmentation of labour with twins is acceptable if indicated. An intravenous infusion should be established and epidural anaesthesia provided as required. Spontaneous or assisted vaginal delivery of the first twin involves the same principles as for a singleton fetus. Additional obstetric and neonatal personnel should be alerted with the anticipation of immediate neonatal care for both twins.[7]

SECOND STAGE OF LABOUR

Many prefer to conduct the second stage in a room where there is the capability of moving straight to caesarean section for those rare cases in which this is needed for the second twin.[8] The availability of ultrasound may help define the lie and presentation of the second twin when there is clinical doubt.

When the first twin is delivered, its cord should be securely clamped in case there is a vascular connection which would allow the second twin to bleed through the cord of the first. After delivery of the first twin there is usually a diminution in uterine contractions. It is therefore advisable at this time to set up an intravenous infusion with five units of oxytocin in 500 ml crystalloid 'piggy-backed' onto the main intravenous line.

As in much of intrapartum care, good judgement is required to achieve a balance between excessive intervention, leading to hurried and traumatic delivery, and passive delay, which might end with asphyxia. This endeavour is aided by careful fetal heart rate monitoring of the second twin.

TECHNICAL ASPECTS OF INTERNAL VERSION AND BREECH EXTRACTION

- With appropriate anaesthesia and uterine relaxation, the forewaters should not be tense and one will be able to feel the parts of the fetus.

- Keeping the membranes intact, grasp one or preferably both feet and pull steadily downwards and backwards into the vagina (Figure 12.1). The relaxed uterus and cushion of amniotic fluid ensure that the fetus converts readily from transverse to breech.

- As you continue traction the membranes will rupture, but by this stage the breech is well on its way to the introitus having being buffered from trauma by the amniotic fluid during its descent. Continue traction until the scapula appears.

- Carry out the remainder of the delivery as outlined in chapter 11.

- When reaching through the membranes for the foot, it is obviously important not to confuse the foot with the hand. The foot is best identified by the point of the heel. One can practise this by feeling the hands and feet of newborn infants with one's eyes closed during other normal births. It is preferable to grasp both feet, but if only one can be reached it is better if it is the anterior foot. If one has grasped the posterior foot, the anterior buttock may arrest on the pubic symphysis during traction. If this occurs, the posterior leg should be rotated 180° in a wide arc during traction to convert it to the anterior position. In these cases the second leg will be extended and can be brought down in the same manner as the extended leg of a frank breech.

If there is intrapartum bleeding, cord prolapse, a non-reassuring fetal heart rate pattern or continued delay despite oxytocin augmentation, delivery should be accelerated. The options include assisted vaginal

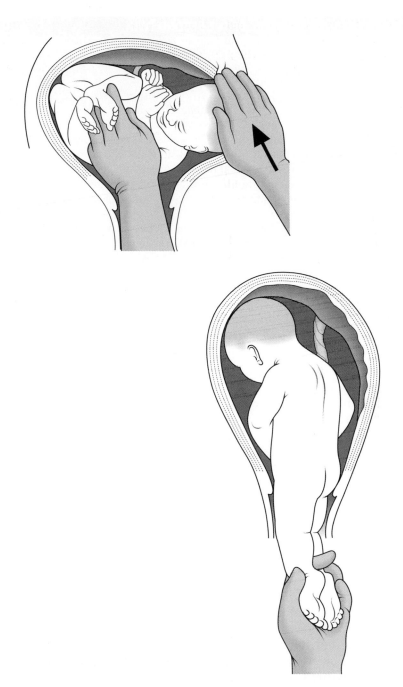

Figure 12.1 Internal version and breech extraction

GUIDELINES FOR DELIVERY OF THE SECOND TWIN

Once the first twin has been delivered, check the lie and presentation of the second twin. If the presentation is cephalic or breech, this pole is steadied at the pelvic brim with one hand while a pelvic examination rules out cord presentation. The 'piggy-backed' oxytocin infusion is started at about 10 drops/minute and titrated to achieve adequate uterine contractions (three to four every 10 minutes of 40–60 seconds' duration). When contractions are regular and the presenting part is stable and descending, the membranes are ruptured. Usually, the fetus will descend with a few contractions to spontaneous or assisted vaginal delivery.

If the second twin is a transverse or oblique lie, external cephalic or podalic version should convert the lie to longitudinal and allow one to proceed as above.

If the second twin is a footling breech or transverse lie, particularly if the transverse lie does not respond to external version, a case can be made for immediate internal version and/or breech extraction. This is one of the few valid indications for these procedures in modern obstetrics. As mentioned in the section on anaesthetic factors (page 147), uterine relaxation is essential before these manoeuvres are considered. A well-relaxed uterus, along with the recent passage of the first twin, creates ideal conditions for this form of delivery.

delivery with forceps or vacuum for cephalic presentations, breech extraction or caesarean section.[8] The choice will depend on the available facilities, anaesthesia, the experience of the accoucheur and the lie and station of the second twin.

An outline of the intrapartum management of the most common combinations in twin pregnancy is shown in Figure 12.2.

Locked twins

Locked twins are extremely rare, occurring in about 1/1000 twin deliveries. However, the risk of lethal asphyxia and trauma, particularly to the first twin, is high. The most likely occurrence is with relatively small fetuses when twin A is breech and twin B vertex (Figure 12.3). In most obstetric units nowadays, twins with this presentation at the start of labour would undergo caesarean section. When locked twins are encountered, it is usual for the first twin breech to deliver normally up to the trunk but for delivery of the shoulders and descent of the arms and head to be arrested. On occasions, under deep general anaesthesia and with uterine relaxation, one can elevate the body of the first twin and disimpact the head of the second twin. This allows one to proceed

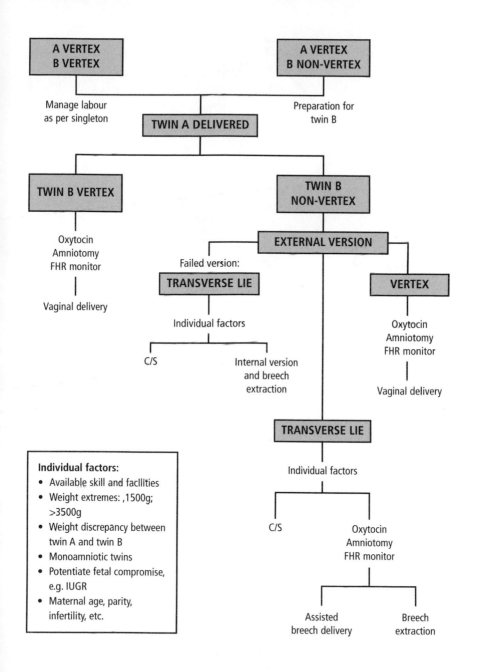

Figure 12.2 Intrapartum management of twin pregnancy

Adapted from: Baskett TF. *Essential Management of Obstetric Emergencies.*
4th ed. Bristol: Clinical Press, 2004.

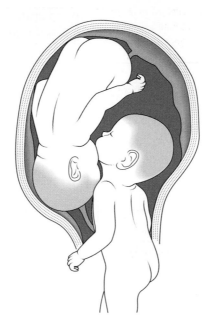

Figure 12.3 Locked twins: breech/vertex

with breech delivery of the first twin and deal with the second twin in the usual manner.[9] If, however, gentle attempts at disimpaction fail, one is usually committed to delivery by caesarean section. This will usually entail a generous classical incision in the uterus to allow 'reverse extraction' of the first twin through the uterine incision, followed by the second twin.

THIRD STAGE OF LABOUR

After delivery of twins, the overdistended uterus is more prone to atony. Thus, active management of the third stage of labour should be followed by an extended (6–8-hour) intravenous infusion of oxytocin.

Triplets and higher-order births

With the use of ovulation-induction agents and assisted reproductive techniques, triplets and higher-order births have increased ten-fold in most developed countries over a 25-year period.[1,10] In many units the majority of, if not all, viable triplets are delivered by elective caesarean section. In addition to obviating the need for experienced and skilled intrauterine and vaginal manipulation, another advantage is to allow the scheduling of three teams for immediate neonatal care. It is also difficult to monitor the fetal heart rates of triplets in labour. However, the risks of caesarean section to the mother are greater and there is no evidence that there is clear benefit to the infants from abdominal versus vaginal delivery. Indeed, recent work suggests that vaginal delivery of triplets at or after 32–34 weeks of gestation may hold some advantages for the infants.[11,12]

Vaginal delivery may be considered in selected cases at or after 32 weeks of gestation if the first triplet is in cephalic presentation and there are no signs of fetal compromise in any of the triplets. Once the first triplet has been born, the next two should be delivered without delay. If they present by the vertex, the membranes can be ruptured and spontaneous or low assisted delivery carried out. If not, immediate internal version and/or breech extraction, with the same safeguards as outlined for the second twin, should be undertaken.[13]

For quadruplets and above, planned caesarean section will be chosen for viable pregnancies.

References

1. Van Voorhis BJ. Outcomes from assisted reproductive technology. *Obstet Gynecol* 2006;107:183–200.
2. American College of Obstetricians and Gynecologists Committee on Practice Bulletins—Obstetrics; Society for Maternal-Fetal Medicine; ACOG Joint Editorial Committee. ACOG Practice Bulletin #56: Multiple gestation: complicated twin, triplet, and high-order multifetal pregnancy. *Obstet Gynecol* 2004;104:869–83.
3. Petterson B, Nelson KB, Watson L, Stanley F. Twins, triplets, and cerebral palsy in births in Western Australia in the 1980s. *BMJ* 1993;307:1239–43.
4. Yokoyama Y, Shimizu T, Hayakawa K. Prevalence of cerebral palsy in twins, triplets and quadruplets. *Int J Epidemiol* 1995;24:943–8.
5. Armson BA, O'Connell C, Persad V, Joseph KS, Young DC, Baskett TF. Determinants of perinatal mortality and serious neonatal morbidity in the second twin. *Obstet Gynecol* 2006;108:556–66.
6. Hack KE, Derks JB, Schaap AH, Lopriore E, Elias SG, Arabin B, et al. Perinatal outcome of monoamniotic twin pregnancies. *Obstet Gynecol* 2009;113:353–60.
7. Benachi A, Pons JC. Is the route of delivery a meaningful issue in twins? *Clin Obstet Gynecol* 1998;41:31–5.
8. Persad VL, Baskett TF, O'Connell CM, Scott HM. Combined vaginal–cesarean delivery of twin pregnancies. *Obstet Gynecol* 2001;98:1032–7.

9. Saad FA, Sharara HA, Locked twins: a successful outcome after applying the Zavanelli manoeuvre. *J Obstet Gynaecol* 1997;17:366–7.
10. Cassell KA, O'Connell CM, Baskett TF. The origins and outcomes of triplet and quadruplet pregnancies in Nova Scotia: 1980 to 2001. *Am J Perinatol* 2004;21:439–45.
11. Dommergues M, Mahieu-Caputo D, Mandelbrot L, Huon C, Moriette C, Dumez Y. Delivery of uncomplicated triplet pregnancies: is the vaginal route safer? A case–control study. *Am J Obstet Gynecol* 1995;172:513–17.
12. Wildschut HI, van Roosmalen J, van Leeuwen E, Keirse MJ. Planned abdominal compared with planned vaginal birth in triplet pregnancies. *Br J Obstet Gynaecol* 1995;102:292–6.
13. Dommergues M, Mahieu-Caputo D, Dumez Y. Is the route of delivery a meaningful issue in triplets and higher order multiples? *Clin Obstet Gynecol* 1998;41:25–9.

13 Caesarean section

Caesarean section has become the most common operation in women owing to the worldwide increase in caesarean delivery rates since the 1980s. A variety of factors have lowered the threshold for performing caesarean section:

- improvements in anaesthesia, blood transfusion, antibiotics, surgical techniques and thromboprophylaxis have combined to increase the safety of caesarean section
- a combination of social and medico-legal expectations of the perfect perinatal outcome
- less experience and an unwillingness to accept even small increased risks associated with certain types of operative vaginal delivery
- changing maternal demographics: increasing maternal age, obesity and reduced parity
- increasing maternal age, infertility and assisted reproductive techniques have led to a rise in the number of so-called 'premium' pregnancies as well as an increase in twin and triplet pregnancies
- improved neonatal care and outcomes have lowered the gestational age at which caesarean section is appropriate for fetal indications
- an uncommon but emerging indication is women requesting elective caesarean section for the perceived benefits of eliminating rare fetal risks in labour and the sequelae of pelvic floor damage to themselves.[1]

Indications

While the indications and their proportion may vary from country to country and hospital to hospital, the big four indications account for 60–90% of all caesarean sections:

- repeat caesarean section (35–40%)
- dystocia (20–35%)
- breech (10–15%)
- fetal distress (10–15%).

In many cases the indication is a combination of dystocia and potential fetal compromise in a non-progressive labour associated with a non-reassuring fetal heart rate pattern. These indications are discussed in their respective chapters.

Analysis of caesarean delivery rates can be readily achieved using the universally applicable Robson 10-group method.[2,3] This consistently shows that the biggest contributor to the caesarean delivery rate is dystocia in the apparently low-risk group of nulliparous women with a single, cephalic fetus at term in spontaneous labour, and particularly in those with induced labour.[3,4] The other major groups leading to caesarean delivery are breech presentation at term and repeat caesarean section. Thus, if reducing the caesarean section rate is a priority, efforts should be concentrated on the management of labour in women having their first baby at term. Additional priorities would be effective measures to reduce breech presentation at term by external cephalic version and the provision of safe facilities for vaginal birth after caesarean section. The increasing contribution of multiple pregnancies to the rising caesarean section rate could be reduced by a more disciplined approach to assisted reproductive techniques with the return of fewer embryos.

General considerations

ANAESTHESIA

Anaesthesia for caesarean section should be regional (epidural or spinal) in the vast majority of cases. Exceptions requiring general anaesthesia may be:

- woman's preference (rare)
- need for speed (acute fetal distress)
- possibility of prolonged surgery, such as uterine rupture or placenta praevia accreta.

ANTIBIOTICS

Prophylactic antibiotics are indicated in all but elective caesarean sections with intact membranes. Some obstetricians will give an antibiotic to all women undergoing a caesarean delivery in an attempt to minimise febrile morbidity. A single intravenous dose, given at cord clamping, of a first-generation broad-spectrum antibiotic such as ampicillin or cephalosporin is effective. In cases with risk factors, such as prolonged labour with ruptured membranes or when there are clinical signs of early chorioamnionitis, the antibiotic may be continued for 24–48 hours.

THROMBOPROPHYLAXIS

After emergency caesarean section, all women should receive graduated compression stockings and low-molecular-weight heparin – the latter for up to 7 days.[5] If there are additional risk factors, the heparin may be continued for longer. Women undergoing elective caesarean deliveries should also receive heparin if there are any additional risk factors for thromboembolism.[5]

Types of caesarean section

LOWER TRANSVERSE SEGMENT CAESAREAN SECTION

Lower transverse segment caesarean section is the type of operation performed in about 98% of cases. The uterine incision is confined to the relatively non-contractile lower uterine segment so that healing is optimal and potential disruption less likely in a subsequent labour.

LOW VERTICAL CAESAREAN SECTION

Low vertical caesarean section has been advocated by some when the lower segment is well developed by advanced labour but, because of earlier gestational age, the width of the lower segment is deemed inadequate to deliver the fetus atraumatically through a transverse incision. This incision also obviates the risk of trauma to the uterine vessels. Should the incision require enlargement, it can be extended vertically into the upper uterine segment to achieve delivery of the fetus. In fact, many so-called low vertical incisions do extend into the upper uterine segment and have at least some of the same drawbacks as the classical incision. Thus, this type of incision is rarely performed and usually only by enthusiastic advocates.

CLASSICAL CAESAREAN SECTION

Classical caesarean section accounts for 1–2% of all caesarean sections in most obstetric units. This rate has increased as the gestational age at which caesarean section is performed has fallen. The vertical incision in the upper uterine segment has the disadvantage of being more vascular and the healing in the puerperium may be disrupted in this contractile portion of the uterus. As outlined in chapter 14, the subsequent rupture of this scar in another pregnancy carries a much higher risk.

The most common indication for classical caesarean section is caesarean section in the earlier weeks of gestation when inadequate formation of the lower uterine segment precludes safe and atraumatic delivery of the fetus through that site. It is also necessary when access to the lower uterine segment is prohibited by uterine fibroids, extensive adhesions and the massive vascularity rarely associated with some cases of major placenta praevia and placenta praevia accreta.

In the vast majority of cases, a lower transverse incision can be planned and performed. In women at earlier gestations, particularly below 34 weeks, and if there has been no labour, the lower segment may not be adequately formed to allow delivery of the fetus through an incision in that site. The final decision can be taken only when the abdomen is opened and the lower segment is inspected directly. As the advantages of the lower transverse incision are considerable, in some marginal cases one starts with this incision but accepts, if there is difficulty in delivering the fetus, that an additional vertical incision – either a J extension into the upper segment on one side or the inverted T in the midline – may have to be performed.[6] In many such cases one can safely perform the lower transverse incision and save the woman the subsequent risks of a classical incision. In those women in whom one has to resort to the J or inverted T incision, the surgical end result is no worse and maternal and perinatal morbidity are not increased compared with a classical incision.[7]

Figure 13.1 shows the different types of caesarean section.

Surgical aspects

LOWER TRANSVERSE SEGMENT CAESAREAN SECTION

As with all operations, individual surgeons develop their own points of technique. However, the following general guidelines seem reasonable.

To avoid aortocaval compression by the uterus, the woman should be placed with a lateral tilt of 15°.

In the majority of all types of caesarean section, the Pfannenstiel incision or modification thereof is adequate and appropriate.[8] The main indication for a lower midline incision is speed of entry for acute fetal compromise or in cases where both speed and extra surgical space may be required, such as uterine rupture.

A urethral Foley catheter should be inserted preoperatively and may be retained for a few hours or overnight following the procedure. During labour, the bladder is elevated and, unless empty, is even more vulnerable to incision during entry to the peritoneal cavity. For this reason the peritoneum is first incised as high as possible and extended down under transillumination.

Once the peritoneal cavity has been opened, check the uterus for dextro- or laevorotation. It is more common to find dextrorotation

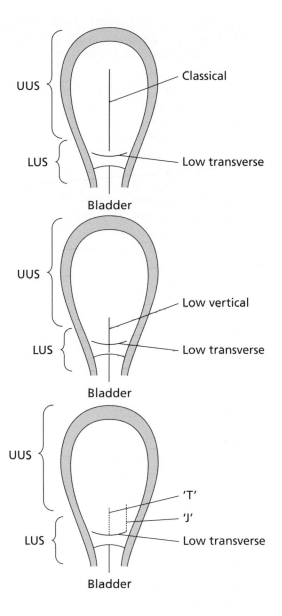

UUS = Upper uterine segment

LUS = Lower uterine segment

Figure 13.1 Caesarean section: types of uterine incision

owing to the sigmoid colon. This has important implications for placement of the incision in the uterus. If this point is ignored, it is easy to make the transverse incision in an eccentric manner such that the uterine vessels are breached on one side.

The uterovesical peritoneum is identified and incised, and with the forefinger the areolar tissue between the lower uterine segment and bladder gently separated. A Doyen, DeLee or Balfour retractor is then placed to move the bladder down safely from the line of uterine incision.

Be aware that in prolonged labour with disproportion, the lower uterine segment may be very stretched and drawn up to form a considerable portion of the lower uterus. In such cases, if the uterine incision is made too low, one risks entering the vagina. Careful attention to the point of reflection from the uterus of the uterovesical peritoneal fold will help with the appropriate placement of the uterine incision.

The initial incision into the uterus must be performed with great care if laceration of the fetus is to be avoided, particularly in cases of obstructed labour with a thin lower segment to which the fetal head is closely applied.[9] Using the scalpel in the midline, a horizontal 2 cm incision is made with very light pressure such that only a few fibres are incised. Sweep the other index finger across this initial incision so that the layers can be seen with precision. Often only two or three very gentle strokes are required to go through the full thickness of the thin lower segment muscle. When partially through the muscle, press and release the centre of the incision with the forefinger: this should raise a 'bleb' of the very thin final layer so that it can be incised without risk to the underlying fetus. Alternatively, use the forefinger or handle of the scalpel to stretch the incision and separate the few remaining muscle fibres to gain entry with blunt dissection. Once the uterus is entered, the forefinger is placed between the fetus and the uterine muscle towards one side and the incision is continued with either curved Mayo or bandage scissors. The same is repeated on the other side. After the initial entry incision, the lateral extensions should be directed upwards so that the final incision is a 'smile' of the 'Cheshire-cat' variety. About 80% of the incision is made with the scissors and then each forefinger is hooked into the angles, so the final extension of the incision is carried out with a pull of each forefinger. In cases in which the width of the lower segment is marginal, the angles of the incision may be directed almost vertically, producing an enlarged 'trapdoor' effect.

If the fetus is in cephalic presentation, manual delivery of the head will usually be adequate. This entails inserting the flat of the lower hand without the thumb between the lower part of the incision and the fetal head. If the head is deeply engaged in the pelvis, it may take considerable effort to elevate it up into the incision. It is important not to use a 'shoehorn' motion to achieve this as you risk extension of the uterine incision down into the vagina. Using the upper hand to grasp the wrist of the lower hand will often aid in elevation and reduce the amount of shoehorn motion. Once the head is elevated into the uterine incision, it is flexed to produce the smallest diameter, following which sustained fundal pressure by the assistant should deliver the head through the uterine and abdominal wall incisions. If there is difficulty, and in some cases where the head is free and floating, forceps or the vacuum can be used to assist delivery of the head.

In the case of breech presentation, the uterine incision is made in the same manner. As outlined in chapter 11, the manoeuvres required for safe delivery of the breech are the same whether by the vaginal route or through a uterine incision. For all cases of breech delivery by caesarean section, and particularly for those at less than 36 weeks of gestation, the anaesthetist should have intravenous glyceryl trinitrate drawn up and ready to administer should head entrapment occur. This is a very real risk with the small breech, the body of which delivers easily through the lower segment while the larger after-coming head may become trapped, particularly with regional anaesthesia when there is no additional uterine relaxation. It is in these cases that the judicious administration of intravenous glyceryl trinitrate can assist atraumatic delivery of the fetal head (see chapter 23, page 245).

For the fetus in transverse lie, delivery through a lower segment incision may, in some cases, be safely undertaken if the membranes are intact and the fetus can be turned to cephalic or breech presentation. Here again, intravenous glyceryl trinitrate may help to achieve this. If successful version has been performed, one has to decide whether the lower segment is sufficiently developed to allow this type of caesarean section or whether one has to move to the classical incision.

Once the head of the infant is safely delivered, the anaesthetist should give five units of oxytocin intravenously, followed by an oxytocin infusion. Once separated, the placenta is delivered by controlled cord traction. After the placenta is delivered, the uterine cavity should be explored for remnants of placenta or membranes. This can be aided by use of a moistened gauze sponge over the hand.

It is inappropriate to routinely perform manual removal of the placenta as this is associated with greater blood loss, potential for infection and even occasional uterine inversion.[10] Unless the placenta is retained, manual removal at the time of caesarean section has no advantages.

Similarly, there is no reason to routinely bring the uterus out of the abdominal incision after delivery of the fetus and placenta. This can cause pain, nausea and vomiting in women under regional anaesthesia.

Even for those with basic surgical skills, there is adequate exposure to repair the uterine incision without this manoeuvre. On the other hand, if there is extension of the uterine incision or heavy bleeding that limits exposure, one should not hesitate to exteriorise the uterus. The ovaries and tubes can be checked without delivering the uterus through the incision.

Before closing the uterine incision, Green-Armytage or ring forceps can be used to compress bleeding sinuses in the muscle edges. Even if there are no bleeds, it is useful to place one forceps to identify the lower edge of the uterine incision. On occasions, the lower edge may be obscured by blood and the posterior wall of the uterine segment may buckle forward and mimic, to the unwary, the lower edge of the uterine incision.

Traditionally, closure of the uterine incision has been in two layers. However, a number of obstetricians have moved to single-layer closure, which saves about 4 minutes of operating time. However, all of the previous literature on labour after caesarean section is based on two-layer closure. There is inadequate, and so far conflicting, data to say whether single-layer closure will have a greater, lesser or similar degree of scar integrity in a subsequent labour.[11-13] The 2010 CAESAR trial showed no difference in short-term infectious morbidity between single-layer and double-layer closure.[14] However, we must await the outcome in subsequent pregnancies before we can conclusively recommend single-layer closure. Furthermore, the largest observational study found subsequent scar rupture to be almost four-fold greater with single-layer compared with double-layer closure.[13] Until there is definitive evidence, the authors recommend two-layer closure.

The first layer is closed with a running suture including the cut edge of uterine muscle and not the decidua. The use of a continuous running suture is best for the first layer as this avoids the bunched-up tissues of a locked suture and facilitates the second-layer closure. After the first layer is inserted, pressure with a pack across the incision with one hand and uterine massage of the fundus with the other will compress the incision line and reduce bleeding. It is common for the upper uterine edge of the incision to be much thicker than the lower. Hence, the second layer of sutures should raise a fold of muscle on the lower side, about 1 cm from the incision, and the same on the upper side, including any unstitched muscle edge. In this manner the first layer of sutures is covered. The second layer can be closed with running or locking sutures, depending on haemostasis. In cases where there is sufficient upper and lower muscle thickness, such as primary elective caesarean section, the inner two-thirds can be stitched as the first layer followed by the outer third as the second layer. The assistant should keep good tension on the suture but not so much as to strangle or cut through the muscle. Most commonly 0 or No, 1 polyglactin (Vicryl) or polyglycolic acid (Dexon) sutures are used for the uterine incision.

Since the late 1990s there has been a recent trend not to close the uterovesical peritoneum and there are some data to support this.[15,16] The CAESAR trial found no difference in postoperative infectious morbidity with closure or non-closure of the visceral peritoneum.[14] However, a study in 2005 showed that peritoneal closure significantly reduces adhesions found at subsequent caesarean section.[17] For closure of the abdominal wall, there is now evidence that the parietal peritoneum need not be closed.[16] It is reasonable to loosely approximate the medial edges of the rectus muscles with two or three interrupted and lightly tied sutures. The rectus sheath is closed with a running suture and it is helpful to lock every third or fourth stitch. No sutures need be placed in the fat tissue: the less foreign material in the wound, the less potential for infection. For skin closure staples, interrupted sutures or a subcuticular suture can be used. All caesarean sections are at least potentially contaminated with the rich bacterial vaginal flora. The advantage of interrupted sutures or staples is that serum can ooze out and is not sealed under the skin incision as a bacterial culture medium. If there is infection, one or two sutures can be removed to allow drainage, whereas with subcuticular sutures the entire area is sealed and drainage is impossible. The long-term cosmetic effect of subcuticular versus interrupted wound skin staples or stitches is the same.

CLASSICAL CAESAREAN SECTION

The entry into the peritoneal cavity for classical caesarean section is the same as for the lower-segment operation. With retraction, the vertical incision in the upper uterine segment can be made through a Pfannenstiel incision. The uterine incision is made with the scalpel starting in the upper part of the lower segment where the uterine wall is thin. Upon entry into the uterus, the rest of the incision is extended upwards by 10–12 cm with scalpel and scissors while the fingers protect the fetal parts. The lower limit of the incision is at the uterovesical peritoneal reflection. If the placenta is encountered under the incision, pass the hand to the nearest placental edge and, if necessary, enlarge the incision to deliver the fetus. Once the fetus and placenta are delivered, it is usual to exteriorise the uterus for closure of the vertical incision. This is a much more vascular incision and it is very helpful to have access to the uterus so that the assistant's hands can encircle the incision with the fingers on one side and the thumbs on the other to compress the incision, assisting its closure and reducing blood loss (Figure 13.2).

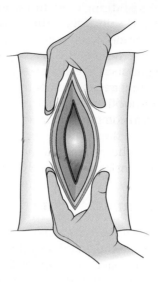

Figure 13.2 Assistant's hands encircle the classical caesarean incision to reduce blood loss and facilitate closure

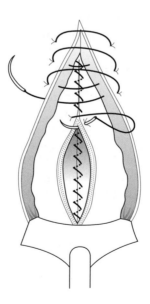

Figure 13.3 Closure of classical incision: the deep layers require two to three continuous running sutures and a final broad locking suture of the seromuscular layer

The uterine incision is closed in two or three layers. The first one or two layers, depending on the thickness of the muscle, are closed using a running suture to bring the deeper layers of uterine muscle together. When the deeper layers have been closed, such that the depth of incised uterine muscle not closed is about 1 cm, the final seromuscular layer is placed. This involves suturing approximately 1 cm from the edge of the incision with a continuous locking suture (Figure 13.3). The role of the assistant is very important in compressing the line of the incision both to reduce blood loss and to take the pull off the sutures as they are placed, so they do not cut through the muscle and allow the locking suture to be applied without undue tension.

LOW VERTICAL CAESAREAN SECTION

Low vertical caesarean section requires greater dissection of the bladder from the lower uterine segment to accommodate the vertical incision. Beware of dissecting off the bladder too much in the lateral aspects or you will excite much bleeding.

The initial vertical entry incision should be made with the same cautionary principles as the lower transverse incision. With a finger protecting the fetal presenting part, the incision is extended up and down with scissors. The main problem is a balance between extending too far downwards into the vascular vagina and too far up into the upper uterine segment. Once the incision is made, the lower end can be stitched and held as a stay suture. This helps prevent extension of the incision into the bladder and vagina, as well as delineating the lower edge to facilitate closure of the uterine wound.

The principles of uterine closure are the same as for the transverse incision.

THE DEEPLY ENGAGED FETAL HEAD

There is increased maternal and neonatal morbidity in caesarean sections performed at full cervical dilatation with a deeply engaged fetal head.[18] Much of this morbidity is attributable to the difficulty of elevating the fetal head that is moulded and deeply impacted in the pelvis. In particular, lateral or downward extensions of the transverse uterine incision, associated with strong shoehorn movements of the surgeon's hand trying to elevate the fetal head, can lead to profuse bleeding in hard-to-isolate areas.

There are three approaches to this dilemma:

- At the time the bladder is catheterised, a vaginal examination is performed and the fetal head pushed up higher in the pelvis.

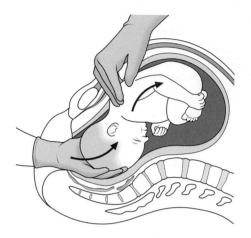

Figure 13.4 Elevation of the deeply engaged fetal head

- At the time of the caesarean section, an assistant cups the fetal head in the palm of their hand and elevates the head while the surgeon puts some manual traction on the fetal shoulders (Figure 13.4). Once the head is sufficiently elevated, the surgeon's hand is inserted below the fetal head in the usual manner for assisted manual delivery.

- The third option is to perform reverse breech extraction.[19–21] The assistant's hand may still try and help elevate the fetal head while the surgeon reaches up into the uterus, grasps the fetal feet and pulls down to deliver the baby by internal version and breech extraction. The body tends to flex and come through the uterine incision, while the fetal head automatically follows up into the space created in the pelvis. The after-coming head is delivered with the same care as for assisted breech delivery. This can be a less traumatic option for both the maternal tissues and the fetus.

POSTOPERATIVE DOCUMENTATION

Finally, a surgical report should be written including the indications for and a description of the operation. In particular, details of extensions of the uterine incision or encroachment into the upper uterine segment will help those involved in a subsequent pregnancy to make reasoned decisions about the next delivery. During the postoperative hospital stay, a review of the above factors with the woman should also take place.

References

1. Declercq E, Menacker F, MacDorman M. Rise in "no indicated risk" primary caesareans in the United States, 1991–2001: cross sectional analysis. *BMJ* 2005;330:71–2.
2. Robson MS, Scudamore IW, Walsh SM. Using the medical audit cycle to reduce cesarean section rates. *Am J Obstet Gynecol* 1996;174:199–205.
3. Robson MS. Classification of caesarean sections. *Fetal Matern Med Rev* 2001;12:23–39.
4. Allen VM, Baskett TF, O'Connell CM. Contribution of select maternal groups to temporal trends in rates of caesarean section. *J Obstet Gynaecol Can* 2010;32:633–41.
5. Royal College of Obstetricians and Gynaecologists. *Reducing the risk of thrombosis and embolism during pregnancy and the puerperium.* Green-top Guideline No. 37a. London: RCOG, 2009 [http://www.rcog.org.uk/womens-health/clinical-guidance/reducing-risk-of-thrombosis-greentop37a].
6. Boyle JG, Gabbe SG. T and J vertical extensions in low transverse cesarean births. *Obstet Gynecol* 1996;87:238–43.
7. Patterson LS, O'Connell CM, Baskett TF. Maternal and perinatal morbidity associated with classical and inverted T cesarean sections. *Obstet Gynecol* 2002;100:633–7.
8. Stark M, Finkel A. Comparison between the Joel Cohen and Pfannenstiel incisions in caesarean section. *Eur J Obstet Gynaecol Reprod Biol* 1994;53:121–2.
9. Alexander JM, Leveno KJ, Hauth J, Landon MB, Thom E, Spong CY, et al.; National Institute of Child Health and Human Development Maternal-Fetal Medicine Units Network. Fetal injury associated with caesarean delivery. *Obstet Gynecol* 2006;108:885–90.
10. Basku A, Kalan A, Ozkan A, Baksu B, Tekelicoglu M, Goker N. The effect of placental removal method and site of uterine repair on postcesarean endometritis and operative blood loss. *Acta Obstet Gynecol Scand* 2005;84:266–9.
11. Chapman SJ, Owen J, Hauth JC. One- versus two-layer closure of a low transverse cesarean: the next pregnancy. *Am J Obstet Gynecol* 1997;89:16–18.
12. National Collaborating Centre for Women's and Children's Health. *Caesarean section. Clinical Guideline.* London: RCOG Press; 2004 [http://www.nice.org.uk/CG013].
13. Bujold E, Bujold C, Hamilton EF, Harel F, Gauthier RJ. The impact of single-layer or double-layer closure on uterine rupture. *Am J Obstet Gynecol* 2002;186:1326–30.
14. CAESAR study collaborative group. Caesarean section surgical techniques: a randomised factorial trial (CAESAR). *BJOG* 2010;117:1366–76.
15. Nagele F, Karas H, Spitzer D, Staudach A, Karasegh S, Beck A, et al. Closure or nonclosure of the visceral peritoneum at cesarean delivery. *Am J Obstet Gynecol* 1996;174:1366–70.

16. Luzuy F, Irion O, Beguin F. Nonclosure of the visceral and parietal peritoneum at caesarean section: a randomised controlled trial. *Br J Obstet Gynaecol* 1996;103:690–4.
17. Lyell DJ, Caughey AB, Hu E, Daniels K. Peritoneal closure at primary cesarean delivery and adhesions. *Obstet Gynecol* 2005;106:275–80.
18. Allen VM, O'Connell CM, Baskett TF. Maternal and perinatal morbidity of caesarean delivery at full cervical dilatation compared with caesarean delivery in the first stage of labour. *BJOG* 2005;112:986–90.
19. Fong YF, Arulkumaran S. Breech extraction – an alternative method of delivering a deeply engaged head at cesarean section. *Int J Obstet Gynecol* 1997;56:183–4.
20. Levy R, Chernomoretz T, Appelman Z, Levin D, Or Y, Hagay ZJ. Head pushing versus reverse breech extraction in cases of impacted fetal head during cesarean section. *Eur J Obstet Gynecol Reprod Biol* 2005;121:24–6.
21. Chopra S, Bagga R, Keepanasseril A, Jain V, Kalra J, Suri V. Disengagement of the deeply engaged fetal head during caesarean section in advanced labor: conventional method versus reverse breech extraction. *Acta Obstet Gynecol Scand* 2009;88:1163–6.

14 Vaginal birth after caesarean section

Since the 1980s, caesarean section rates have risen worldwide. In many developed countries, one-quarter to one-third of all pregnant women have a caesarean delivery, while 10–12% of the obstetric population have been previously delivered by caesarean section. Thus, about one in ten pregnant women, and those looking after them, have to consider the implications for pregnancy, labour and delivery after previous caesarean section. The main consideration is the balance between the risks and benefits of elective repeat caesarean section versus trial for vaginal birth after caesarean section.

Selection

The most dreaded complication is, of course, uterine rupture (chapter 15). Thus, a trial for vaginal delivery can be contemplated only when the appropriate personnel and facilities are available. Anaesthesia, nursing and obstetric staff should be immediately available together with the appropriate operating facilities and blood transfusion. These issues have been reviewed in national society guidelines.[1–3]

The principle of informed consent is very important in these women. Women should understand the maternal risks involved with caesarean section, both elective and after failed trial for vaginal delivery. The possibility of complete uterine rupture in labour (approximately 3–6/1000) should be presented together with the risk of perinatal death and/or severe morbidity should rupture occur: about 1–2/1000 more than with repeat elective caesarean delivery.[3,4]

The previous obstetric chart should be reviewed for details of the indication for, type and perioperative course of the previous caesarean delivery. The following factors will form the basis for evaluation of risk and the discussion leading to informed consent:

- Type of uterine scar:
  - Classical caesarean section scars will rupture in 4–9% of subsequent pregnancies: about 10 times more often than a lower

uterine segment scar. Furthermore, the upper-segment scar is more likely to rupture before labour, in contrast to lower-segment scar rupture, which usually occurs after some hours of labour when the woman is in hospital and prompt treatment is available.

o Hysterotomy scars, like classical caesarean scars, are a contra-indication to subsequent labour.

o Low vertical caesarean section is not often performed, but when undertaken is it is performed in early gestation when the lower uterine segment is not sufficiently developed to allow a transverse incision. Despite its name, the incision often encroaches on the upper uterine segment and in a subsequent pregnancy is best treated as a classical scar.

o Extension of the uterine incision beyond one or both angles requires individual consideration based on the operation report. T and J incisions are best not subjected to labour.

o Myomectomy incisions, either open or via hysteroscopy, may be vulnerable to rupture if they are extensive, and particularly if they involved the full thickness of the myometrium.

o Previous uterine rupture is a contraindication to labour.

• Previous vaginal delivery: vaginal delivery before or after the previous caesarean section is the single most reliable predictor of a successful trial and vaginal delivery in a subsequent pregnancy.[5,6]

• Timing of previous caesarean section: the timing of the previous caesarean section in labour is an important guide to the type of uterine strain and work required in the next pregnancy.[7] Thus, a woman who had a previous caesarean section, either with no labour or in the latent phase of labour, will exhibit the stronger pattern of uterine work similar to that of the nulliparous woman. By contrast, the woman with a previous caesarean section in the active phase of labour (fully effaced cervix, greater than 3 cm dilatation) will show a multiparous pattern of labour with less uterine work and less strain on the uterine scar.

• Previous caesarean section for dystocia: if the previous caesarean section was for dystocia, the chance of successful subsequent vaginal delivery is reduced but not enough to preclude a trial if other factors are favourable.

• More than one previous caesarean section: women who have had more than one previous lower transverse segment caesarean section may labour and deliver successfully, but the risk of uterine rupture is increased and the woman should be aware of this.[8]

• Uterine incision closure: there is conflicting evidence regarding an increased risk of subsequent scar rupture if the previous caesarean myometrial closure was single layer compared with double layer.[9,10] Large randomised trials are under way that should answer this question. In the meantime, neither technique precludes a trial of vaginal delivery.

• Postcaesarean infection: postpartum endometritis may interfere with caesarean scar healing and increase the risk of subsequent rupture.[11] In the clinical context, many postcaesarean fevers are attributable to causes other than endometritis. If there is good clinical evidence that the infection was uterine, a subsequent labour is best avoided.

• Inter-pregnancy interval: an inter-pregnancy interval of less than 18 months may be associated with a higher risk of uterine scar disruption.[3,12]

• Twin pregnancy: the woman with twins in the next pregnancy is a controversial candidate for trial of vaginal delivery, not least because there are two fetuses at potential risk. Overdistention of the uterus with twins and the possibility of intrauterine manipulation for delivery of the second twin increases the potential risk of rupture in this group, although success has been reported.[13,14]

• Lower uterine segment thickness: preliminary studies suggest that ultrasonographic measurement of the lower uterine segment may help select those with a higher risk of scar rupture.[15,16] Further work is needed to delineate the clinical role of this promising approach.

• Neonatal respiratory morbidity: respiratory distress and transient tachypnoea of the newborn are increased with elective caesarean section without labour. This can be kept to a minimum, and of minimal severity, by booking the repeat caesarean at no earlier than 39 weeks of gestation.[3]

• Cumulative risks of repeated caesarean deliveries: women should be aware of the increased risks of severe morbidity in the form of placenta praevia accreta, injury to the lower urinary tract and the potential need for hysterectomy with increasing numbers of repeat caesarean deliveries. For women having up to three caesareans, the risk is less than 2%.[17]

Consideration of the combination of the above factors should allow the woman and her doctor to make a reasonably informed decision. Coercion, subtle or otherwise, is inappropriate. The discussion leading to informed consent should be carefully documented in the chart. There is much to be said for a hospital-based information brochure for women considering vaginal birth after caesarean section, which could serve as a consistent starting point for the discussion.

Management

ANTENATAL CARE

Apart from a detailed review of the factors noted above, antenatal care should be routine.

INDUCTION OF LABOUR

Spontaneous labour is always preferable to induced labour and only well-established indications for induction should be considered. While there may be a compelling reason for induction, the woman should be informed that this increases, by two- to three-fold, the risk of uterine rupture and its sequelae.[3] This risk is lowest with oxytocin after amniotomy and higher if prostaglandins are used.[18–21] The use of misoprostol for induction of labour is associated with an unacceptable rate of uterine rupture and misoprostol should not be used for this purpose.[22,23]

Thus, in any case in which induction of labour is considered, the obstetrician should pose the question: 'Why am I not performing a caesarean section?' It may be that the woman wants to have more pregnancies and to avoid the risks of multiple caesareans. If, however, she is having only one more pregnancy, the additional risks of induction may not be justified. Furthermore, successful vaginal birth after caesarean section is less likely when labour is induced rather than spontaneous.

The spectrum of clinical presentation may also guide this decision, from women with a favourable cervix, in whom amniotomy and oxytocin alone would likely be effective, to those with a cervix of carrot-like consistency, in whom repeated doses of prostaglandins have to be considered.

LABOUR

A plan should be in place and documented in the chart for the 10% of women booked for elective repeat caesarean section who go into labour before 39 weeks of gestation.

The woman with a previous caesarean section should be advised to come into hospital early in labour. Blood should be taken for group and screen. In the early stages, if all is normal, it is reasonable to allow the woman to ambulate. Once labour is established, it is prudent to insert an intravenous drip. Epidural analgesia may be provided as indicated for any other labour. The theoretical worry that epidural might mask the pain and tenderness of uterine rupture has not been substantiated. Continuous electronic fetal heart monitoring is advised, as one of the earliest signs of uterine dehiscence is abnormality of the fetal heart rate.

The progress of labour should be carefully charted using a partogram. To be safe, one should expect a normal progressive labour. Although one tries to manage the labour in as normal a manner as possible, this is not a normal labour and the risks to the mother and infant are increased. Discretion is usually the better part of valour if labour is non-progressive.

Oxytocin augmentation of non-progressive labour should be considered only in hospitals with on-site obstetric and anaesthesia personnel and women should be informed that oxytocin augmentation increases the risk of uterine rupture. If augmentation is undertaken, one should anticipate a smooth progressive response; if this does not occur, a repeat caesarean section should be performed.

SIGNS AND SYMPTOMS OF UTERINE RUPTURE

The clinical presentation of uterine rupture can vary from mild and non-specific to an obvious abdominal catastrophe. The picture of catastrophic uterine rupture with sudden severe lower abdominal pain, cessation of uterine contractions, vaginal bleeding, dramatic elevation of the presenting part, fetal death and signs of intra-abdominal haemorrhage is rare with rupture of a low transverse caesarean scar. The transverse lower segment scar is thin and avascular and may dehisce with minimal or even no clinical signs, only to be discovered postpartum or as a surprise finding at caesarean section performed for reasons other than suspected uterine rupture. That said, the lower segment scar can rupture with rapidly progressive compromise and death of the fetus.

The following signs and symptoms of early uterine rupture can be inconsistent but are nonetheless valuable in the early detection of rupture:

- The most consistent and reliable sign of early uterine rupture is abnormality of the fetal heart rate. This may include tachycardia or variable and late decelerations, with prolonged bradycardia being the most worrying sign.

- Persistent pain and tenderness over the lower uterine segment between uterine contractions is another sign of early uterine rupture. It can be hard to interpret as a minor degree of these symptoms may exist in normal labour. Continuous and worsening point tenderness should not be ignored.

- In the thin woman, central or unilateral swelling and crepitus over the lower uterine segment may be detected.

- The bladder is often adherent to the site of the lower segment caesarean scar such that the integrity of the bladder wall may be breached if the uterine scar gives way, leading to haematuria and, occasionally, tenesmus. In this context, haematuria may be one of the more important early warning signs of uterine rupture.

● There may be no, a little or a lot of vaginal bleeding. The caesarean scar is avascular and may give way with no bleeding. If, however, the rupture extends beyond the scar, there may be heavy bleeding, although this may be confined to the peritoneal cavity.

● Maternal hypotension, tachycardia and syncope may occur with the associated intraperitoneal bleeding.

There has been no large randomised trial to compare vaginal birth after caesarean section with elective repeat caesarean section, but there is considerable published evidence to support vaginal birth after caesarean section in selected women.[3] However, the rare catastrophic clinical and medico-legal sequelae associated with uterine rupture and with survival of a severely compromised infant has led to a considerable reduction in the offer and acceptance of planned vaginal birth after caesarean section in many countries.[24] A meta-analysis of studies from the 1990s suggests a slightly increased risk of the rare events of uterine rupture and neonatal morbidity and mortality with a trial for vaginal delivery, and an increased rate of maternal morbidity with elective caesarean section.[25]

As with many areas of medicine, the problem is the 'pendulum syndrome', when excessive zeal in attempts to achieve vaginal delivery leads to unreasonable risk. With careful selection, the majority of women will have a smooth and progressive labour, achieving vaginal delivery with minimal risk to themselves and the infant. When additional risk factors and interventions are added, the risk of scar rupture increases with very little gain in the number of vaginal deliveries achieved. This is yet another area of obstetrics where sensible clinical balance is required.

References

1. American College of Obstetricians and Gynecologists. ACOG Practice Bulletin No. 115: Vaginal birth after previous cesarean delivery. *Obstet Gynecol* 2010;116:450–63.
2. Martel MJ, MacKinnon CJ; Clinical Practice Obstetrics Committee, Society of Obstetricians and Gynaecologists of Canada. Guidelines for vaginal birth after previous Caesarean birth. *J Obstet Gynaecol Can* 2005;27:164–88.
3. Royal College of Obstetricians and Gynaecologists. *Birth after previous caesarean birth*. Green-top Guideline No. 45. London: RCOG; 2007 [http://www.rcog.org.uk/womens-health/clinical-guidance/birth-after-previous-caesarean-birth-green-top-45].

4. Smith GC, Pell JP, Cameron AD, Dobbie R. Risk of perinatal death associated with labor after previous cesarean delivery in uncomplicated term pregnancies. *JAMA* 2002;287:2684–90.

5. Zelop CM, Shipp TD, Repke JT, Cohen A, Lieberman E. Effect of previou vaginal delivery on the risk of uterine rupture during a subsequent trial labor. *Am J Obstet Gynecol* 2000;183:1184–6.

6. Gyamfi C, Juhasz G, Gyamfi P, Stone JL. Increased success of trial of labc after previous vaginal birth after cesarean. *Obstet Gynecol* 2004;104:715–9

7. Arulkumaran S, Gibb DM, Ingemarsson I, Kitchener HS, Ratnam SS. Uterine activity during spontaneous labour after previous lower-segment caesarean section. *Br J Obstet Gynaecol* 1989;96:933–8.

8. Bretelle F, Cravello L, Shojai R, Roger V, D'ercole C, Blanc B. Vaginal birth following two previous cesarean sections. *Eur J Obstet Gynecol Reprod Biol* 2001;94:23–6.

9. Bujold E, Bujold C, Hamilton EF, Harel R, Gauthier RJ. The impact of single-layer or double-layer closure on uterine rupture. *Am J Obstet Gynecol* 2002;186:1326–30.

10. Durnwald C, Mercer B. Uterine rupture, perioperative and perinatal morbidity after single-layer and double-layer closure at cesarean delivery. *Am J Obstet Gynecol* 2003;189:925–9.

11. Shipp TD, Zelop C, Cohen A, Repke JT, Liebermann E. Post-cesarean delivery fever and uterine rupture in a subsequent trial of labour. *Obstet Gynecol* 2003;101:136–9.

12. Bujold E, Mehta SH, Bujold C, Gauthier RJ. Interdelivery interval and uterine rupture. *Am J Obstet Gynecol* 2002;187:1199–202.

13. Guise JM, Hashima J, Osterweil P. Evidence-based vaginal birth after Caesarean section. *Best Pract Res Clin Obstet Gynaecol* 2005;19:117–30.

14. Ford AA, Bateman BT, Simpson LL. Vaginal birth after cesarean delivery in twin gestation: a large, nationwide sample of deliveries. *Am J Obstet Gynecol* 2006;195:1138–42.

15. Rozenberg P, Goffinet F, Philippe HJ, Nisand I. Thickness of the lower segment: its influence in the management of patients with previous cesarean sections. *Eur J Obstet Gynecol Reprod Biol* 1999;87:39–45.

16. Jastrow N, Chaillot N, Roberge S, Morency AM, Lacasse Y, Bujold E. Sonographic lower uterine segment thickness and risk of uterine scar defect: a systematic review. *J Obstet Gynaecol Can* 2010;32:321–7.

17. Silver RM, Landon MB, Rouse DJ, Leveno KJ, Spong CY, Thom EA, et al.; National Institute of Child Health and Human Development Maternal-Fetal Medicine Units Network. Maternal morbidity associated with multiple repeat cesarean deliveries. *Obstet Gynecol* 2006;107:1226–32.

18. Landon MB, Hauth JC, Leveno KJ, Spong CY, Leindecker S, Varner MW, et al.; National Institute of Child Health and Human Development Maternal-Fetal Medicine Units Network. Maternal and perinatal outcomes associated with a trial of labor after prior cesarean delivery. *N Engl J Med* 2004;351:2581–9.

19. Smith GC, Pell JP, Pasupathy D, Dobbie R. Factors predisposing to perinatal death related to uterine rupture during attempted vaginal birth after caesarean section: retrospective cohort study. *BMJ* 2004;329:375.
20. Ravasia DJ, Wood SL, Pollard JK. Uterine rupture during induced trial of labor among women with previous cesarean delivery. *Am J Obstet Gynecol* 2000;183:1176–9.
21. Lydon-Rochelle M, Holt VL, Easterling TR, Martin DP. Risk of uterine rupture during labor among women with a prior cesarean delivery. *N Engl J Med* 2001;345:3–8.
22. Wing DA, Lovett K, Paul RH. Disruption of prior uterine incision following misoprostol for labor induction in women with previous cesarean delivery. *Obstet Gynecol* 1998;91:828–30.
23. Plaut MM, Schwartz ML, Lubarsky SL. Uterine rupture associated with the use of misoprostol in the gravid patient with a previous cesarean section. *Am J Obstet Gynecol* 1998;180:1535–42.
24. Yeh J, Wactawski-Wende J, Shelton JA, Reschke J. Temporal trends in the rates of trial of labor in low-risk pregnancies and their impact on the rates of vaginal birth after cesarean delivery. *Am J Obstet Gynecol* 2006;194:144–8.
25. Mozurkewich EL, Hutton EK. Elective repeat cesarean delivery versus trial of labor: a meta-analysis of the literature from 1989 to 1999. *Am J Obstet Gynecol* 2000;183:1187–97.

15 Uterine rupture

The hospital incidence of uterine rupture varies from 1/100–500 deliveries in developing countries to 1/1000–5000 deliveries in countries with well-developed hospital services.[1-3]

The type of rupture may be complete, involving the full thickness of the uterine wall, with or without extrusion of fetal parts, or incomplete, when the uterine muscle has separated but the visceral peritoneum remains intact. Excluding separation of previous uterine scars, the most common site of complete rupture is the anterior lower uterine segment. Uterine rupture may extend laterally with bleeding into the broad ligament and retroperitoneal space. Less common is rupture of both the distended lower segment and the vaginal fornix. In 5–10% of cases, the rupture involves the bladder wall.

In regions with poorly developed obstetric services, the maternal mortality rate can reach 10–20% and the perinatal death rate 40–90%.[2-4] Although maternal death owing to uterine rupture is uncommon in developed countries, the morbidity for the mother can be high, and can include the need for hysterectomy.[5] In addition, perinatal morbidity as a result of hypoxic–ischaemic encephalopathy is a risk with well-developed services, where the relatively rapid performance of caesarean section may diminish the risk of stillbirth only to salvage a severely hypoxic infant.[6]

Causes

UTERINE SCAR

Rupture of a previous caesarean section scar is by far the most common cause of uterine rupture in developed countries, accounting for about 90% of all cases.[7] Scars that encroach on the upper uterine segment are more prone to rupture because this contractile part of the uterus may disrupt healing of the scar during the puerperium. In addition, during a subsequent labour the upper uterine segment contracts actively compared with the more passive lower segment. Estimates of uterine rupture associated with pregnancy and labour vary as follows: classical incision 4–9%, low vertical incision 1–7% and low transverse incision 0.2–1.5%. Details of this cause of uterine rupture are covered in chapter 14.

Although there is less experience, hysterotomy incisions seem to behave in the same manner as classical caesarean section. Myomectomy scars that are not large and do not involve the full thickness of the uterine wall are less prone to rupture.[8] However, those that are extensive, particularly if they involve the full thickness of the uterine wall, are more vulnerable to dehiscence.

Other events that may scar and weaken the uterine wall to a greater or lesser degree include: uteroplasty, salpingectomy with deep cornual resection, previous uterine perforation, repeated and extensive curettage and operative hysteroscopy.[8] Deep cervical scars associated with conisation, amputation and cerclage may risk rupture if they encroach on the lower uterine segment.

OBSTRUCTED LABOUR

Obstructed labour is the most common cause of uterine rupture in developing countries. The main predisposing factors are cephalopelvic disproportion, malpresentations such as transverse lie, and fetal anomalies such as hydrocephalus.[9] The multiparous uterus is most vulnerable to uterine rupture as it often responds to obstruction with stronger uterine contractions, whereas the nulliparous uterus will tend to react with diminished uterine activity. In this context, oxytocin augmentation of non-progressive labour in the multiparous woman should be undertaken with considerable caution.

Rupture of the unscarred nulliparous uterus is extremely rare and usually found only with uterine anomalies or with excessive use of oxytocin or misoprostol.[10–12]

TRAUMA

Obstetric uterine trauma should be extremely rare in well-run maternity services but may be caused by internal version and breech extraction, forceps rotation, fetal destructive operations, shoulder dystocia and manual removal of an accretic placenta. Traumatic laceration of the uterus can occur in association with surgical termination of pregnancy in the first 20 weeks. External trauma, such as a motor vehicle accident, stab wounds or gunshot, is a relatively rare cause.

MISCELLANEOUS

There are a number of rare specific conditions that can predispose to uterine rupture, such as:

- uterine anomalies
- gestational trophoblastic disease
- placenta accreta, increta and percreta
- cornual pregnancy
- severe concealed placental abruption.

In general, the multiparous uterus is much more vulnerable to uterine rupture because repeated pregnancy leads to fibrosis and thinning of the uterine muscle. The clinical features of uterine rupture may vary from an obvious intra-abdominal haemorrhagic catastrophe to very mild and non-specific signs, as outlined in chapter 14.

Management

Treat hypovolaemia with intravenous crystalloid and blood products as necessary.

Perform laparotomy and remove the fetus and placenta. It is essential to rapidly secure haemostasis; to achieve this, the uterus is brought up out of the incision. The assistant's hands are placed behind the uterus and, with the thumbs and index fingers at each side, the uterine vessels can be compressed. The extent of the uterine rupture can then be delineated and the bleeding edges occluded with Green-Armytage or ring forceps.

If uterine conservation is desirable, bilateral uterine and ovarian artery ligation may be swiftly performed (see chapter 19).

If the uterine laceration is simple and the desire for future reproduction strong, it may be acceptable just to repair the laceration, provided haemostasis is secured.[13,14] In these cases, good results can be achieved when subsequent pregnancies are delivered by elective caesarean section.[15] Alternatively, repair of the rupture and tubal ligation may be appropriate.

In all cases, the procedures should be covered by perioperative anti-biotics and the integrity of the bladder wall should always be checked.

Many patients with uterine rupture will require hysterectomy, which is considered in chapter 16.

References

1. Pettersson KW, Grunewald C, Thomassen P. Uterine rupture and perinatal outcome. *Acta Obstet Gynecol Scand* 2007;86:1337–41.
2. Sahin HG, Kolusari A, Yildizhan R, Kurdoglu M, Adali E, Kamachi M. Uterine rupture: a twelve-year clinical analysis. *J Matern Fetal Neonatal Med* 2008;21:503–6.

3. Gardeil F, Daley S, Turner MJ. Uterine rupture in pregnancy reviewed. *Eur J Obstet Gynecol Reprod Biol* 1994;56:107–10.
4. Mishara SK, Morris N, Uprety DK. Uterine rupture: preventable obstetric tragedies? *Aust N Z J Obstet Gynaecol* 2006;46:541–5.
5. Turner MJ. Uterine rupture. *Best Pract Res Clin Obstet Gynaecol* 2002;16:69–80.
6. Martinez-Biarge M, García-Alix A, García-Benasach F, Gayá F, Alarcón A, González A, et al. Neonatal neurological morbidity associated with uterine rupture. *J Perinat Med* 2008;36:536–42.
7. Kieser KE, Baskett TF. A 10-year population-based study of uterine rupture. *Obstet Gynecol* 2002;100:749–53.
8. Dow M, Wax JR, Pinette MG, Blackstone J, Cartin A. Third-trimester uterine rupture without previous cesarean: a case series and review of the literature. *Am J Perinatol* 2009;26:739–44.
9. Aboyeji AP, Ijaiya MD, Yahaya UR. Ruptured uterus: a study of 100 consecutive cases in Ilorin, Nigeria. *J Obstet Gynaecol Res* 2001;27:341–8.
10. Miller DA, Goodwin TM, Gherman RB, Paul RH. Intrapartum rupture of the unscarred uterus. *Obstet Gynecol* 1997;89:671–3.
11. Lang CT, Landon MB. Uterine rupture as a source of obstetrical hemorrhage. *Clin Obstet Gynecol* 2010;53:237–51.
12. Walsh CA, Baxi LV. Rupture of the primigravid uterus: a review of the literature. *Obstet Gynecol Surv* 2007;62:327–34.
13. Soltan MH, Khashoggi T, Adelusi B. Pregnancy following rupture of the pregnant uterus. *Int J Gynaecol Obstet* 1996;52:37–42.
14. Al-Sakka M, Hamsho A, Khan L. Rupture of the pregnant uterus – a 21-year review. *Int J Gynaecol Obstet* 1998;63:105–8.
15. Lim AC, Kwee A, Bruinse HW. Pregnancy after uterine rupture: a report of 5 cases and a review of the literature. *Obstet Gynecol Surv* 2005;60:613–7.

16 Emergency obstetric hysterectomy

Emergency postpartum hysterectomy is one of the most commonly accepted markers of severe maternal morbidity.[1] The incidence varies from about 1/350 to 1/7000 deliveries and the maternal mortality rate ranges from 0% to 35%.[2–4] The higher incidence and mortality rates are found in regions with limited hospital resources. In developed countries the incidence of emergency obstetric hysterectomy is about 1/2000–3000.[5–7] There is an association between emergency hysterectomy and caesarean section[6,8,9] and between emergency hysterectomy and multiple pregnancy.[10–12] With increasing rates of caesarean delivery and with assisted reproductive techniques producing more multiple pregnancies, the need for obstetric hysterectomy is increasing in some countries. For example, in Canada between 1991 and 2003 the obstetric hysterectomy rate rose significantly from 0.26/1000 deliveries to 0.46/1000 deliveries.[13]

Indications

The three main conditions leading to obstetric hysterectomy are abnormal placentation, uterine atony and uterine rupture and trauma.[9,14–17]

ABNORMAL PLACENTATION: PLACENTA PRAEVIA AND/OR ACCRETA

The rising incidence of delivery by caesarean section has been accompanied by an increased risk of placenta praevia and/or accreta in subsequent pregnancies, making these the most common reasons for obstetric hysterectomy in developed countries.

UTERINE ATONY

Uterine atony is the second most common reason for obstetric hysterectomy. Although prostaglandins have been added to the oxytocic drugs available for the management of uterine atony, there are still occasions when the uterus is refractory to all uterotonic agents. This is

...ticularly so in cases of prolonged labour with clinical or subclinical ...rioamnionitis, where the exhausted and infected uterus may not ...ond to uterotonic drugs.

...RINE RUPTURE AND TRAUMA

...he most common cause of uterine rupture is a previous caesarean scar, and the rising caesarean delivery rates contribute to this cause. Other less common reasons are the inappropriate use of oxytocic drugs in the first and second stage of labour and trauma associated with obstetric manipulation, such as internal version and breech extraction.

The above three reasons account for more than 90% of obstetric hysterectomies in developed countries. Other causes include sepsis, secondary postpartum haemorrhage, recurrent uterine inversion and cornual and cervical ectopic pregnancies.

Surgical aspects

The surgical technique for obstetric hysterectomy is similar to that for abdominal hysterectomy in gynaecological cases, with some modifications to account for the considerable anatomical and physiological changes of pregnancy. The main surgical principles are described below.[18]

Subtotal hysterectomy may be chosen if the cervix and paracolpos are not involved in the rupture or haemorrhagic site. Subtotal hysterectomy is simpler, faster and less likely to injure the lower urinary tract than total hysterectomy. In many cases, subtotal hysterectomy is a good example of surgical discretion being the better part of valour. Total hysterectomy is required if the cervix or paracolpos is involved as the source of bleeding, or if there is marked sepsis.

Many of the pedicles are very thick, oedematous and vascular. Therefore, they should be doubly clamped and ligated. To avoid haematoma formation, place a free tie proximally and a second transfixing suture distal to the free tie. Pedicles are more likely to remain secure if they are smaller, placed in the correct anatomical plane (avoid twisting) and have a generous tissue pedicle distal to the ligature. To avoid the ureter, after clamping the uterine arteries, place all other clamps medially.

When performing a total hysterectomy it can be quite difficult to identify the cervix, particularly if it has reached full dilatation. The process can be made easier by placing a finger down through the uterine incision into the vagina and hooking it up to identify the rim of the cervix. The vagina should then be entered posteriorly and the incision carefully guided laterally and anteriorly.

In many instances of uterine rupture, the integrity of the bladder wall is vulnerable. This is particularly so in cases of ruptured lower-segment scars, to which the bladder is often adherent. In most cases, therefore, it is appropriate to test the integrity of the bladder wall intraoperatively with dye or sterile milk inserted through the Foley catheter. Sterile milk is preferable: it is easily obtained from the nursery and does not stain the tissues. Thus, it is easier to check the integrity of the bladder repair with repeat instillation. Any tear in the bladder should be repaired in two layers using 3/0 polyglactin or similar suture.

In cases with extensive bladder laceration requiring repair, or with haemostatic sutures needed in the paracolpos, there may be doubt about the integrity of the ureters. If so, it is advisable to perform a post-operative cystoscopy to observe the efflux of urine from each ureteric orifice. If necessary, this can be aided by giving intravenous indigo carmine 10–15 minutes beforehand.

Perioperative antibiotics should be continued for at least 48 hours. Postoperative thromboprophylaxis should be instituted.

It is ideal to identify potential damage to the bladder or ureters and correct it at the time of operation, both for clinical reasons and for litigation defence. If lower urinary tract injuries are not diagnosed until the postoperative period, the clinical morbidity and diagnostic and surgical management are more complex and prolonged; this is also associated with increased litigation vulnerability.[19] Thus, if it is feasible in the context of the emergency circumstances, any lower urinary tract injury should be sought and dealt with at the time of the hysterectomy.

In some cases after hysterectomy there may be continued bleeding from the pelvic basin. This is usually due to the development of disseminated intravascular coagulation leading to oozing from the traumatised tissues despite ligation of obviously bleeding pedicles. In these cases the application of a pelvic pressure pack may be life-saving, either providing permanent haemostasis or stemming the flow sufficiently until additional haematological, surgical or vessel embolisation resources can be made available.[20] The pack is assembled by filling a plastic bag with gauze rolls tied together, such that the base of the bag has a broad area that will fill the pelvic basin. This narrows at the neck of the bag which is passed through the vaginal vault from above (Figure 16.1). Either a gauze bandage or intravenous tubing is tied to the neck of the pack and attached to a bag of intravenous fluid which acts as a traction weight suspended over the foot of the bed. In this way the pressure of the pack is distributed over the soft tissues and tamponade achieved against the firm fascia and bones of the pelvis (Figure 16.2). The gauze can be removed slowly and incrementally from below, followed by the collapsed plastic bag.

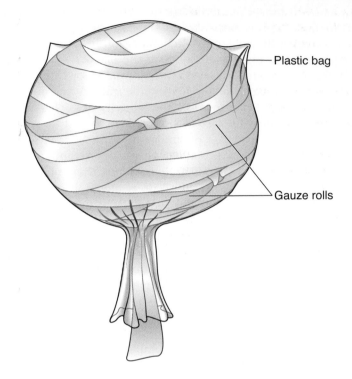

Figure 16.1 Components of pelvic pressure pack

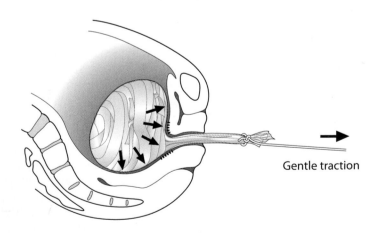

Figure 16.2 Pelvic pressure pack in place

After such a potentially catastrophic event as obstetric hysterectomy, detailed perioperative notes should be placed in the chart. These should include the sequence of events and the rationale for the decisions taken. Reference should be made to the fact that the integrity of the lower urinary tract was checked. A debriefing session of all involved staff is advisable.

Morbidity associated with hysterecomy

The morbidity associated with obstetric hysterectomy is considerable and includes blood transfusion, disseminated intravascular coagulation, operative damage to the bladder and ureters and sepsis.[6,17] In many series approximately 25% of these women require intensive care. Maternal death, although uncommon in countries with sophisticated medical services, is common in those with limited resources. In up to 25% of cases the woman may be primiparous with the associated fertility-ending implications.[6]

Obstetric hysterectomy is undertaken only after other conservative measures, usually to control haemorrhage, have been tried and failed. Elsewhere in this book are described a number of conservative measures including the use of oxytocic drugs, uterine tamponade, uterine compression sutures and major vessel ligation and embolisation. The balance between the use of these techniques and the definitive hysterectomy to control haemorrhage can be a major test of obstetric judgement. If excessive delay is involved, with the ineffectual application of conservative measures, the woman may descend into disseminated intravascular coagulation so that by the time hysterectomy is undertaken it is too late and the outcome is fatal. The prompt and decisive use of conservative measures is appropriate and the timing of hysterectomy will depend upon their effectiveness and, to some extent, the woman's age, parity and desire for future childbearing.

A detailed review and discussion of events leading up to the hysterectomy should be carried out with the woman and her partner following the event. These women are often 'shell-shocked' by a series of events that starts with an anticipated normal labour and delivery but spirals out of control, ending up with blood transfusion, general anaesthesia superimposed on a regional anaesthetic, a stay in intensive care and the loss of her uterus and fertility. Thus, before discharge from hospital it is essential that an experienced obstetrician sit down with the couple and review events in detail. This should include an expression of sympathy that she has lost her uterus and an apology for all the complications she has faced. This is not an admission that her care was substandard but humane recognition of the traumatic event that she has endured.

For the obstetrician these cases demand a blend of the best of the art and science of obstetric judgement under testing conditions.

References

1. Baskett TF, O'Connell CM. Severe obstetric maternal morbidity: a 15-year population-based study. *J Obstet Gynaecol* 2005;25:7–9.
2. Korejo R, Jafarey SN. Obstetrics hysterectomy – five years experience at Jinnah Postgraduate Medical Centre, Karachi. *J Pak Med Assoc* 1995;45:86–8.
3. Yamamoto H, Sagae S, Nishikawa S, Kudoo R. Emergency postpartum hysterectomy in obstetric practice. *J Obstet Gynaecol Res* 2000;26:341–5.
4. Ezechi OC, Kalu BK, Njokanma FO, Nwoloro CA, Okeke GC. Emergency peripartum hysterectomy in a Nigerian hospital: a 20-year review. *J Obstet Gynaecol* 2004;24:372–3.
5. Englesen IB, Albrechtsen S, Iverson OE. Peripartum hysterectomy – incidence and maternal morbidity. *Acta Obstet Gynecol Scand* 2001;80:409–12.
6. Baskett TF. Emergency obstetric hysterectomy. *J Obstet Gynaecol* 2003;23:353–5.
7. Knight M, Kurinczuk JJ, Spark P, Brocklehurst P; United Kingdom Obstetric Surveillance System Steering Committee. Cesarean delivery and peripartum hysterectomy. *Obstet Gynecol* 2008;111:97–105.
8. Kacmar J, Bhimani L, Boyd M, Shah-Hosseini R, Piepert J. Route of delivery as a risk factor for emergency peripartum hysterectomy: a case–control study. *Obstet Gynecol* 2003;102:141–5.
9. Daskalakis G, Anastasakis E, Papantoniou N, Mesogitis S, Theodora M, Antsaklis A. Emergency obstetric hysterectomy. *Acta Obstet Gynecol Scand* 2007;86:223–7.
10. Walker MC, Murphy KE, Pan S, Yang Q, Wen SW. Adverse maternal outcomes in multifetal pregnancies. *BJOG* 2004;111:1294–6.
11. Francois K, Ortiz J, Harris C, Foley MR, Elliott JP. Is peripartum hysterectomy more common in multiple gestations? *Obstet Gynecol* 2005;105:1369–72.
12. Baskett TF, O'Connell CM. Maternal critical care in obstetrics. *J Obstet Gynaecol Can* 2009;31:218–21.
13. Wen SW, Huang L, Liston R, Heaman M, Baskett TF, Rusen ID, et al.; Maternal Health Study Group, Canadian Perinatal Surveillance System. Severe maternal morbidity in Canada, 1991–2001. *CMAJ* 2005;173:759–64.
14. Sebitloane MH, Moodley J. Emergency peripartum hysterectomy. *East Afr Med J* 2001;78:70–4.
15. Bai SW, Lee HJ, Cho JS, Park YW, Kim SK, Park KH. Peripartum hysterectomy and associated factors. *J Reprod Med* 2003;48:148–52.
16. Sheiner E, Levy A, Katz M, Major M. Identifying risk factors for peripartum cesarean hysterectomy. A population-based study. *J Reprod Med* 2003;48:622–6.

17. Smith J, Mousa HA. Peripartum hysterectomy for primary postpartum haemorrhage: incidence and maternal morbidity. *J Obstet Gynaecol* 2007;27:44–7.

18. Baskett TF. Peripartum hysterectomy. In: B-Lynch C, Keith LG, Lalonde AB, Karoshi M , editors. *A Textbook of Postpartum Haemorrhage: a comprehensive guide to evaluation, management and surgical intervention.* Kirkmahoe: Sapiens; 2006. p. 312–5.

19. Gilmour DT, Baskett TF. Disability and litigation from urinary tract injuries at benign gynaecologic surgery in Canada. *Obstet Gynecol* 2005;105:109–14.

20. Dildy GA, Scott JR, Saffer CS, Belfort MA. An effective pressure pack for severe pelvic hemorrhage. *Obstet Gynecol* 2006;108:1222–6.

17 Cord prolapse

Cord prolapse is the quintessential obstetric emergency. It occurs when part of the umbilical cord descends below the fetal presenting part. If the membranes are intact, the condition is called cord presentation. The frequency range is about 1/200 to 1/600 deliveries. The fetal risk is from hypoxia owing to physical compression of the umbilical cord vessels between the fetal presenting part and maternal tissues, or spasm of the vessels as a result of the colder temperature should the cord prolapse through the introitus. The perinatal mortality rate can be as high as 9%, even in well-equipped hospitals.[1]

Aetiology

FACTORS THAT PREDISPOSE TO CORD PROLAPSE

Fetal
- Preterm labour and low birthweight
- Malpresentations
- Anomaly
- Multiple pregnancy

Placental
- Placenta praevia

Amniotic fluid
- Polyhydramnios
- Prelabour rupture of membranes: spontaneous and amniotomy
- Rupture of membranes in labour: spontaneous and amniotomy

Maternal
- Pelvic tumours, such as cervical fibroid
- Pelvic contraction
- Obstetric manoeuvres: rotation of fetal head, version, amnioinfusion

From the list of factors that predispose to cord prolapse, it can be seen that anything that interferes with the close application of the presenting part to the lower uterine segment and cervix will increase the likelihood of cord prolapse. Many of these factors are interrelated, such as preterm labour, malpresentations, multiple pregnancy and polyhydramnios.[2-5]

The potential for amniotomy to cause cord prolapse is often cited. However, studies have not shown an increased risk of cord prolapse with amniotomy compared with spontaneous rupture of the membranes.[6,7] With a prudent approach to amniotomy for both induction and augmentation of labour, this need not lead to an increased risk of cord prolapse. Indeed, should prolapse of the cord occur at the time of amniotomy, it is more likely to be diagnosed and dealt with promptly compared with cord prolapse occurring at the time of spontaneous rupture of the membranes.

By far the most common predisposing factors are the preterm low-birthweight infant, malpresentations and multiple pregnancy.

Diagnosis

The clinical spectrum of umbilical cord prolapse may vary from the dramatic loop of cord outside the introitus to the more subtle, barely palpable, cord beside and just below the presenting part. The diagnosis is usually made by vaginal examination, which should be carried out to exclude cord prolapse in all cases with specific fetal heart abnormalities in labour (such as bradycardia or marked variable decelerations) and after spontaneous rupture of the membranes associated with breech presentation or a high presenting part.

Cord presentation is a much rarer diagnosis that is sometimes made with a loop of cord felt through the membranes and below the presenting part, or using ultrasound before the onset of or during early labour.[8]

Management

Speed is of the essence and the perinatal outcome is largely dictated by the diagnosis-to-delivery interval. The three components of management are:

• prevent or relieve cord compression and cord artery spasm

• fetal assessment

• prompt delivery of the infant.

PREVENT OR RELIEVE CORD COMPRESSION AND CORD ARTERY SPASM

If the cord has prolapsed outside the introitus, the umbilical circulation is compromised by spasm of the umbilical vessels as a result of the colder temperature. Thus, the cord should be cradled gently in the hand and replaced as high as possible in the vagina. Careful handling of the cord is necessary as even light trauma may also cause spasm of the vessels. When the cord has been replaced in the vagina, or if the cord has prolapsed within the vagina only, the entire cord should be cradled in the palm of the hand in such a manner that the compression forces of the vagina are relieved. The tips of the fingers should elevate the presenting part so that it does not directly compress the cord (Figure 17.1).

Place a Foley catheter in the bladder and fill to tolerance, or approximately 500 ml, which should assist in elevating the presenting part and prevent cord compression.[9,10] This can be particularly helpful if any delay in delivery of the infant is anticipated.

Intravenous tocolytic treatment may have rare application when uterine contractions interfere with cord decompression and delay is incurred (see chapter 23, page 246).

The woman's position should be changed to allow gravity to aid decompression of the cord. If possible, the bed should be put in the Trendelenburg position. Initially, the woman should be placed in the knee–chest position, which gives maximum elevation of the presenting part. If there is any delay, this is too tiring a position to maintain and the

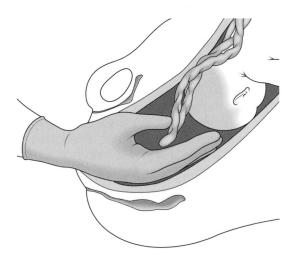

Figure 17.1 Manual protection of cord compression

woman can be moved to the lateral Sims position with the buttocks elevated by pillows.

If facilities for anaesthesia and caesarean section are not immediately available, the above tactics must be maintained and have, on occasions, been applied successfully for several hours. In these cases the lateral Sims position with elevated hips is the most comfortable for the woman and the full bladder technique the most practical for prolonged cord decompression.

Very rarely, with minor degrees of cord prolapse it is possible to replace the cord above the presenting part and allow labour to continue. Occasionally this is easily achieved, but it is not appropriate to attempt too much manipulation as it risks trauma and prolonged vascular spasm of the cord.

FETAL ASSESSMENT

While cord compression is being relieved, urgent attention should be directed to assessing the fetus. If the fetus is dead or immature or has a lethal anomaly, immediate caesarean section is obviously contra-indicated. In many cases the antenatal record will provide information on gestation and the presence or absence of a lethal anomaly. If the woman has no antenatal record, a clinical estimate will have to be made of the size and viability of the infant.

Whether or not the fetus is alive is best determined by listening to the fetal heart rate and/or palpating umbilical artery pulsations. On occasion this can be quite difficult and maternal soft-tissue pulsations may be detectable. In addition, the clinician is often summoned at speed to the labour ward and arrives in a hyperdynamic state, so that pulsations in their own fingers may be confusing.

If there are no detectable pulsations in the cord, a scalp electrode may be of assistance, particularly in monitoring the fetus during the delay between diagnosis and delivery. If available, real-time ultrasound of the fetal chest should confirm the presence or absence of fetal heart activity. Fetal heart activity may be present even in the absence of umbilical artery pulsations, if available, and ultrasound confirmation should be undertaken before abandoning the fetus without detectable cord pulsation.[11]

DELIVERY

In most cases of cord prolapse, the fetus should be delivered by immediate caesarean section. The person whose hand is cradling the cord and elevating the presenting part should remain in position during the induct-

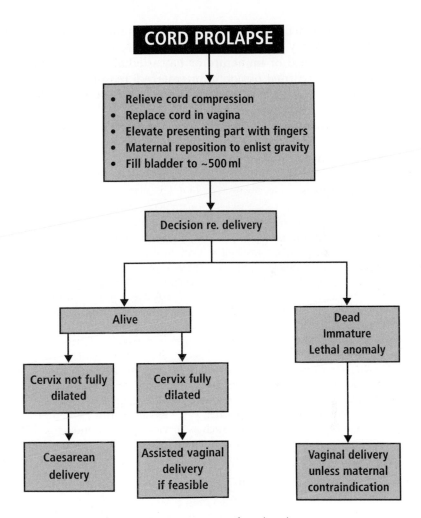

Figure 17.2 Management of cord prolapse

ion of anaesthesia and the placement of sterile sheets. If the full bladder technique has been used, the Foley catheter is drained at this point; if not, a catheter is inserted. Once the caesarean section is under way, and as the surgeon approaches the lower-segment incision, a warning can be issued to remove the protective hand from the surgical site.

In many cases the urgency of the situation requires rapid induction of general anaesthesia. However, if successful cord decompression has been achieved and the fetal heart rate is monitored and stable, the less risky option of spinal anaesthesia may be undertaken.

On rare occasions the cervix is fully dilated and the presenting part low in the pelvis along with the prolapsed cord. In these cases rapid assisted vaginal delivery will be the choice. Depending on the circumstances, this may involve delivery by forceps, vacuum or breech extraction.

If the fetus is dead or immature or has a lethal anomaly, caesarean section would be carried out only for maternal reasons that cannot be resolved safely by vaginal manipulation and delivery, such as an obstructed labour with a transverse lie.

The management of cord prolapse is summarised in Figure 17.2. It is emphasised that in the vast majority of cases the calm and orderly application of the above principles will result in safe delivery of the infant.[12]

References

1. Murphy DJ, MacKenzie IZ. The mortality and morbidity associated with umbilical cord prolapse. *Br J Obstet Gynaecol* 1995;102:826–30.
2. Koonings PP, Paul RH, Campbell K. Umbilical cord prolapse. A contemporary look. *J Reprod Med* 1990;35:690–2.
3. Critchlow CW, Leet TL, Benedetti TJ, Daling JR. Risk factors and infant outcomes associated with umbilical cord prolapse: a population-based case–control study among births in Washington State. *Am J Obstet Gynecol* 1994;170:613–18.
4. Boyle JJ, Katz VL. Umbilical cord prolapse in current obstetric practice. *J Reprod Med* 2005;50:303–6.
5. Lin MG. Umbilical cord prolapse. *Obstet Gynecol Surv* 2006;61:269–77.
6. Ylä-Outinen, Heinonen PK, Tuimala R. Predisposing and risk factors of umbilical cord prolapse. *Acta Obstet Gynecol Scand* 1985;64:567–70.
7. Roberts WE, Martin RW, Roach HH, Perry KG Jr, Martin JN Jr, Morrison JC. Are obstetric interventions such as cervical ripening, induction of labor, amnioinfusion, or amniotomy associated with umbilical cord prolapse? *Am J Obstet Gynecol* 1997;176:1181–3.
8. Jones G, Grenier S, Gruslin A. Sonographic diagnosis of funic presentation: implications for delivery. *BJOG* 2000;107:1055–7.
9. Katz Z, Shoham Z, Lancet M, Blickstein I, Mogilner BM, Zalel Y. Management of labor with umbilical cord prolapse: a 5-year study. *Obstet Gynecol* 1988;72:278–80.
10. Runnebaum IB, Katz M. Intrauterine resuscitation by rapid urinary bladder instillation in a case of occult prolapse of an excessively long umbilical cord. *Eur J Obstet Gynecol Reprod Biol* 1999;84:101–2.
11. Driscoll JA, Sadan O, Van Gelderen CJ, Holloway GA. Cord prolapse – can we save more babies? Case reports. *Br J Obstet Gynaecol* 1987;94:594–5.
12. Royal College of Obstetricians and Gynaecologists. *Umbilical cord prolapse*. Green-top Guideline No. 50. London: RCOG; 2008 [http://www.rcog.org.uk/womens-health/clinical-guidance/umbilical-cord-prolapse-green-top-50].

18 Antepartum haemorrhage

Antepartum haemorrhage is bleeding from the genital tract from 20 weeks of gestation until delivery of the baby. This definition may vary from 20 to 24 weeks of gestation in different countries, in keeping with local medical and legal definitions of fetal viability.

The main causes of antepartum haemorrhage are placenta praevia (1/200–300), placental abruption (1/100) and unclassified (1/100) maternities. In addition, a number of women present with antepartum bleeding from lower genital tract lesions such as vulvovaginal varices, cervical polyps and cervical cancer. While it is important to diagnose and treat such lesions, they will not, as a group, be considered further in this chapter.

Placenta praevia

In placenta praevia, the placenta is implanted in part or in whole on the lower uterine segment, which is that portion of the uterus beneath the reflection of the uterovesical peritoneum. Functionally, it is that part of the myometrium that develops in the latter half of pregnancy, is stretched and thinned during late pregnancy and is relatively passive and non-contractile. When fully developed in labour, it may extend 7–8 cm from the internal os: about the length of the examining finger.

The incidence of placenta praevia is increased with higher parity, advancing maternal age and in those previously delivered by caesarean section; the latter two factors are seen in increasing number in the obstetric population. The overall recurrence risk of placenta praevia is about 1/20.

The classification and terminology of the types or degrees of placenta praevia are as follows:

- type I (lateral or low-lying): extends onto the lower uterine segment but not as far as the edge of the internal os

- type II (marginal): the edge of the placenta extends down to the internal os but does not cover it

- type III (partial): the edge of the placenta covers the internal os but only partially when it is dilated

● type IV (complete or central): the placenta completely covers the cervix even at full dilatation.

Types I and II constitute a minor degree and types III and IV a major degree of placenta praevia.

With modern ultrasound diagnosis there is a tendency to classify placenta praevia simply as minor or major, grouping the original four categories into two. Approximately 50% of all cases of placenta praevia are minor and 50% are major (Figure 18.1).

CLINICAL FEATURES

In the later weeks of pregnancy and during labour, the lower uterine segment is progressively stretched and thinned. It is therefore common for that part of the placenta implanted on the lower uterine segment to separate and cause bleeding. In about 80% of cases this bleeding will occur before the onset of labour. In general, the more major the degree of praevia, the earlier and heavier the bleeding, although some minor degrees can be just as treacherous.

As the bleeding comes from the placental site in the lower uterine segment, there is minimal resistance to the blood passing through the cervix and therefore little or no extravasation of blood into the uterine muscle, resulting in painless bleeding. Consequently, the uterus is usually soft and not tender, and the woman's haemodynamic status corresponds to the apparent blood loss. In contrast to placental abruption, the fetus is rarely threatened by placenta praevia, particularly with the first bleed.

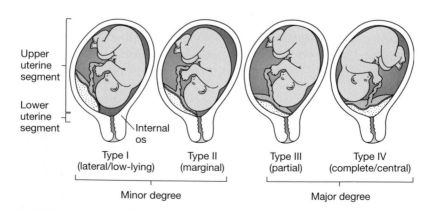

Figure 18.1 Types of placenta praevia

Table 18.1 Clinical features of placental abruption and placenta praevia

Placental abruption	Placenta praevia
May be associated with hypertensive disorders, uterine overdistension, trauma	Apparently causeless
Abdominal pain and/or backache	Painless
Uterine tenderness	Uterus not tender
Increased uterine tone	Uterus soft
Usually normal presentation	Malpresentation and/or high presenting part
Fetal heart may be absent	Fetal heart usually normal
Shock and anaemia out of proportion to apparent blood loss	Shock and anaemia correspond to apparent blood loss

Reproduced with permission from Baskett TF. *Essential Management of Obstetric Emergencies.* 4th ed. Bristol: Clinical Press Ltd; 2004. p. 67

With the placenta occupying part or all of the lower uterine segment, the presenting part of the fetus is more commonly high and free, with malpresentations such as breech, transverse or unstable lie being found in about 40% of cases.

The distinguishing clinical features between placenta praevia and placental abruption are shown in Table 18.1.

DIAGNOSIS

Ultrasound is the diagnostic technique of choice. However, early in the second trimester, when most screening ultrasounds are performed, the lower uterine segment is unformed and extends only 0.5 cm from the internal os. Thus, a false diagnosis of low-lying placenta is commonly made at this stage. With transabdominal ultrasound this may occur in 5–20% of cases, although transvaginal ultrasound has improved considerably upon this level of accuracy. Furthermore, transvaginal ultrasound has not been found to increase the risk of haemorrhage if the placenta is praevia. If an ultrasound diagnosis of possible placenta praevia is made in the second trimester in an asymptomatic woman, ultrasound should be repeated at 32–34 weeks of gestation when the lower segment is formed and the true position of the placenta can be delineated.

The ultimate confirmation of the diagnosis is to feel the placenta with the examining finger placed through the cervix. Such examination is performed only under planned, double set-up conditions. With the accuracy of transvaginal ultrasound this is now rarely necessary, although it may have occasional application under certain circumstances (page 199).

MANAGEMENT

If the woman's ultrasound suggests placenta praevia in the second trimester but there is no bleeding, a repeat ultrasound is planned for 32–34 weeks of gestation to delineate the true site of the placenta (see page 197). In the vast majority of cases, the placenta that is thought to be low-lying in the second trimester will be shown not to be so.

If, at 32–34 weeks of gestation, a transvaginal ultrasound continues to show a minor degree of placenta praevia, the woman should be advised of this and warned to avoid vaginal intercourse, limit her travel and have a mechanism to seek immediate attention if vaginal bleeding occurs. If no bleeding occurs, the woman may be managed as an outpatient until 36–38 weeks of gestation, at which point a repeat ultrasound should be performed. At this point, the woman should be admitted for delivery, which may be by elective caesarean section if the accuracy of ultrasound in the institution is such that the diagnosis of placenta praevia is secure. If there is any doubt, or if there is only a minor degree of placenta praevia, examination in the operating theatre should be arranged to confirm or deny the diagnosis (see page 199).

The asymptomatic woman who has a major degree of placenta praevia at the 32–34-week ultrasound should be admitted to hospital for the remainder of her pregnancy. This remains the safest teaching, which we support. However, there are no conclusive data to support or refute this approach and some will consider close outpatient supervision of these cases if there are compelling social reasons to do so.

The woman who has an antepartum bleed should be admitted, have an intravenous infusion established with crystalloid and have blood taken for group, screen and cross-match. Clinical assessment may then point to the likelihood of placenta praevia or placental abruption. Provided the bleeding is not of a magnitude that requires immediate intervention, ultrasound can be arranged to confirm or deny the diagnosis of placenta praevia. In general, the first bleed associated with placenta praevia settles spontaneously and is not threatening to either the mother or the fetus.

If bleeding occurs before the onset of labour, before 37–38 weeks of gestation, and provided it settles, expectant management is undertaken. This entails keeping the woman in hospital, seeking and treating anaemia and, in selected cases, performing a speculum examination to rule out concomitant lower genital tract lesions. If the patient is rhesus D (RhD)-negative, Rh immune globulin should be given and a Kleihauer test performed to ensure that an adequate dose has been given to cover any fetomaternal bleed. The woman is initially treated with bed rest and bathroom privileges and then allowed more freedom in the ward. In those cases under 34 weeks of gestation, betamethasone to mature the fetal lungs should be considered in case early intervention is necessary.

The cost to the health service and the disruption to the woman and her family of admission to hospital, potentially for several weeks, is considerable. There is controversy as to whether all women with a confirmed diagnosis of placenta praevia should remain in hospital or whether the decision can be made on a selective basis.[1-3] There are no unequivocal data upon which to base this decision. However, in general, those women who have a placenta praevia and bleed before the onset of labour have a worse perinatal outcome than those who do not bleed.[4-6] Thus, if one is going to be selective in admitting women with placenta praevia, those who have bled should be admitted.

If the woman has reached 37–38 weeks of gestation, if labour is established or if the woman continues to bleed, active management in the form of delivery is indicated. If the accuracy of ultrasound in the hospital is unequivocal, delivery will be by caesarean section. If the level of ultrasound is not secure, and in parts of the world where ultrasound may not be available, the so-called double set-up examination in the operating theatre may be necessary. This entails the availability of anaesthesia, nursing personnel and equipment immediately prepared to move straight to caesarean section should the presence of placenta praevia be confirmed by gentle digital examination. First, the fornices are palpated to determine whether the fetal head can be easily felt or if there is a 'boggy' feel suggesting placenta. If the fetal head is easily felt through the fornices, the examining finger is gently passed through the cervix to explore the lower segment. If the placenta is not found to encroach upon the lower uterine segment by the examining finger, amniotomy and careful monitoring of the subsequent labour may be appropriate.

In general, all cases of confirmed placenta praevia are now treated by caesarean section. One can make an argument for amniotomy and careful monitoring of the induced labour in those cases with the most minor degree of praevia, in which the presenting part has settled past the bleeding edge of the placenta and all other aspects are favourable. However, in all but these few cases, caesarean section is more appropriate.

TECHNICAL ASPECTS OF CAESAREAN SECTION FOR PLACENTA PRAEVIA

In most cases, the lower uterine segment is sufficiently developed to allow a low transverse incision to be made. Often there are enlarged vessels over the lower uterus; however, provided the lower segment is well developed, this should not deter one from using the transverse incision. It is also possible to transfix and tie large vessels above and below the line of the intended incision to reduce blood loss. If the lower segment is marginally developed and there are large vessels at the lateral margins, classical caesarean section may be the safer option.

Once the uterine incision has been made in the usual fashion, it is best to go to the edge of the placenta, rupture the membranes and bring the presenting part through the incision. Scrutiny of the ultrasound before the operation should guide the direction, whether this be up, down or lateral, to gain access to the membranes. This is much better than cutting through the placenta, which increases the risk of fetal exsanguination.

Because the lower uterine segment is much less contractile than the upper segment, bleeding from the placental site in this area is common. A number of techniques can be used to try and overcome haemorrhage from the placental site:

- Firm packing of the lower uterine segment for 4 minutes will often reduce the bleeding completely or help delineate specific bleeding sites that can be oversewn with figure-of-eight sutures.

- Alternatively, square sutures through the entire thickness of the uterine wall may help stem oozing areas.[7] Make sure to leave a gap between the sutures to allow egress of the lochia.

- Subendomyometrial injection at multiple sites, each of 1–2 ml solution of vasopressin (five units in 20 ml saline), has been recorded as effective in some cases.[8]

- Application to the lower uterine segment of a pack soaked with Monsel's solution has been used with success in one case series.[9]

- If conservation of the uterus is strongly desired, both uterine arteries can be ligated, although this may not sufficiently reduce the blood supply to the area of the internal os.

- Another option is to provide tamponade with a balloon device and bring this out through the cervix and vagina.[10] The lower uterine segment is then sewn over this balloon. This may be effective when the upper uterine segment is well contracted and the bleeding is coming purely from the placental site in the lower segment. Such treatment may also allow one to buy time and marshal the resources for internal iliac artery embolisation.[11]

If the above is unsuccessful, and particularly if the woman's family is complete, total abdominal hysterectomy should be definitive. In this instance, subtotal hysterectomy may fail to stem the bleeding from the residual lower segment and cervix (see chapter 16).

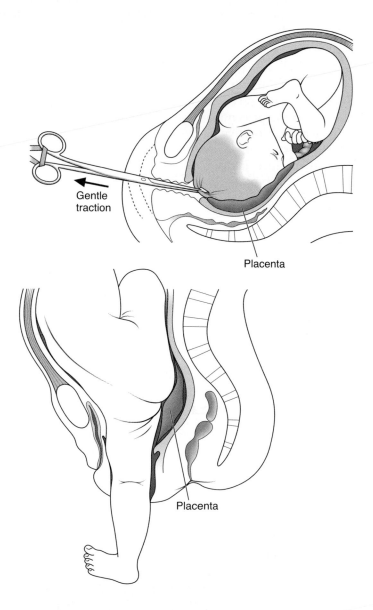

Figure 18.2 Vaginal delivery with placenta praevia

VAGINAL DELIVERY WITH PLACENTA PRAEVIA

There may be rare occasions, such as intrauterine death, lethal anomaly, extreme prematurity or lack of appropriate hospital facilities, when the largely historical techniques of assisted vaginal delivery may be appropriate. Depending on the fetal presentation, there are two procedures[12] (Figure 18.2):

- Braxton Hicks bipolar podalic version: the external hand is applied to guide the breech over the pelvic brim and two fingers of the internal hand are pushed through the cervix to grasp a foot and pull it through the membranes and cervix. In this manner, the fetal buttock acts by tamponade on the placenta and the bleeding lower uterine segment. This can be a very effective haemostat. The fetus is not forcibly pulled through the cervix, but enough steady, gentle traction is applied to the foot to produce tamponade and actively promote progressive dilatation of the cervix. This can be achieved by tying a gauze bandage to the fetal foot and hanging the bandage over the end of the bed tied to a bag of saline.

- Willet's technique: should the fetus present by the head, Willett's technique involves the application of scalp forceps to the fetal head through the incompletely dilated cervix, with traction applying tamponade and assisted delivery in a similar manner to the Braxton Hicks method. Allis forceps or a multitoothed tenaculum can be used for this purpose.

These techniques are very rarely indicated but are worth keeping in mind for the rare case of a dead or non-viable fetus or in places with inadequate facilities for caesarean section.

Placenta praevia accreta

Placenta praevia accreta, one of the most surgically demanding haemorrhagic complications of pregnancy, is relatively rare, occurring in about 1/3000–5000 deliveries. However, the main risk factor, anterior placenta praevia, is increasing as a result of rising caesarean delivery rates.

Histologically, there are three degrees of pathological adherence of the placenta:

- accreta: the plane between the decidua compacta and decidua spongiosa is abolished
- increta: chorionic villi invade the myometrium
- percreta: invasion extends through the myometrium to the serosal surface and sometimes into adjacent organs, particularly the bladder.

In histopathological terms, all three degrees may coexist in a single case. In clinical practice, the general term accreta is used and individual treatment is guided by clinical and surgical findings.

DIAGNOSIS

Placenta accreta should be considered in all cases of placenta praevia, especially anterior placenta praevia in women with a caesarean scar. Ultrasound, using Doppler and power amplitude angiography techniques, is conclusive or highly suggestive. In cases of posterior placenta praevia, magnetic resonance imaging is more accurate.[13] Antenatal diagnosis is desirable so that the appropriate management can be undertaken on an elective rather than an emergency basis.

MANAGEMENT

With a likely or certain diagnosis, preoperative discussion and planning with the appropriate personnel will produce the best results. This may involve anaesthesia, urology or urogynaecology, gynaecological oncology and interventional radiology. Haematology and blood transfusion services should also be notified.[14,15] Preoperative anaemia should be sought and corrected. The woman and her husband should be informed of the implications, including the probable need for hysterectomy and blood transfusion.

In some hospitals, acute normovolaemic haemodilution and cell saver techniques are considered. Another potential pre-emptive move is the placement of vascular balloon catheters in the internal iliac arteries. Immediately after delivery of the baby, the balloons are inflated to occlude the internal iliacs with a view to reducing blood loss during the hysterectomy. The vessels can also be embolised. There are mixed reports on the benefits of this procedure.[16,17]

If there is likely bladder involvement with a percreta, consider preoperative cystoscopy and placement of ureteric stents.

With some or all of the above manoeuvres in place, the operation is planned for 35–38 weeks of gestation, with or without amniocentesis for fetal lung maturity depending on fetal assessment and the presence or absence of bleeding or uterine activity. The aim is to achieve maximum maturity and yet perform the caesarean and additional required surgery in an elective fashion before labour.[18,19]

If there is placenta percreta, a lower midline incision can be chosen to allow for the extra surgical procedures that may be necessary.

A classical incision is made in the uterus, away from the placental site. The baby is delivered and no attempt made to deliver the placenta. The uterine incision is closed for haemostasis and a total hysterectomy is then performed. Because the main haemorrhage site is the lower uterine segment, a subtotal hysterectomy is inadequate (see chapter 16).

If the bladder wall is involved by a percreta, it may be possible to 'shave' off the percretic portion of the uterine wall, leaving a thin layer attached to the bladder. Bleeding from the residual attached area may be stopped by pressure, figure-of-eight sutures or Monsel's solution. Alternatively, if the attached percretic area of the uterus is small, the bladder may be opened and an ellipse of the posterior bladder wall with the attached percreta excised. Care must be taken to ensure that this area does not involve the ureteric orifices when reconstituting the bladder wall.[20]

Conservative surgical treatment of placenta accreta has a small role in women who are desperate to retain their uterus and potential fertility. This involves the classical caesarean as described above. Provided there is no placental separation, there should be no immediate bleeding. Adjunctive techniques may include internal iliac artery embolisation and the use of methotrexate to theroretically aid degeneration of the placenta. There is no evidence of benefit of methotrexate and its adverse effect of bone marrow depression may reduce the mother's defence against infection; as a result, methotrexate has largely been discontinued for this purpose. The conservative approach is fraught with the risks of sepsis and secondary haemorrhage – a potentially lethal combination. In many cases the woman will still lose her uterus, but the hysterectomy will be carried out in emergency conditions with a higher morbidity and mortality. The woman and her husband must be aware of the scale of these risks before embarking on conservative treatment.

There may be a place for more conservative management of partial placenta accreta in the upper uterine segment, including excision of the affected area and reconstruction of the uterus.[19] However, this is rarely applicable to placenta praevia accreta unless the accretic area is small and there is adequate uterine muscle remaining in the lower segment.

Caesarean section for placenta praevia, with or without accreta, is not a procedure for the inexperienced. Senior and experienced staff must be present for these cases as the haemorrhage can be massive and unrelenting.

Vasa praevia

Vasa praevia is an uncommon but potentially disastrous complication that occurs in about 1/3000–5000 deliveries. Vasa praevia is associated with velamentous insertion of the cord, in which the site of umbilical cord insertion is into the membranes rather than directly into the placenta.

Thus, the umbilical vessels pass between the membranes, unsupported by Wharton's jelly, before running into the placenta. These vessels are therefore very vulnerable to compression and tearing. When the vessels of velamentous insertion run across the lower segment and cervix in front of the presenting part, vasa praevia exists. On rare occasions, the vessels can be felt by the astute examiner during pelvic examination.

The vessels may be compressed as the fetal presenting part descends or, more commonly, be torn when the membranes rupture either spontaneously or by amniotomy. If, at the time of rupture of the membranes, there is bleeding and associated fetal heart rate abnormality such as bradycardia or sinusoidal pattern, vasa praevia should be suspected and immediate delivery by caesarean effected. There is usually no time to confirm the fetal origin of the bleeding using the Apt or Kleinhauer tests, although this is an option if the fetal heart is stable.

Unfortunately, the perinatal mortality rate is about 60%, so efforts have been undertaken to make the prenatal diagnosis of vasa praevia. This can be achieved by ultrasound screening of the placental cord insertion followed by transvaginal colour Doppler of those cases with a low-lying placenta or an indistinct placental cord insertion. This approach yields a high perinatal survival rate and therefore prenatal screening for vasa praevia may be justified in cases of low-lying placenta.[16]

Placental abruption

Placental abruption is the partial or complete premature separation of a normally situated placenta before the birth of the fetus. In the older literature it was called 'accidental' haemorrhage to distinguish it from the 'inevitable' haemorrhage of placenta praevia. The incidence of placental abruption is increasing owing to the frequency of the associated conditions listed below. Both maternal and perinatal morbidity and mortality rates are increased. The perinatal mortality rate can be 10–20%, much of which is associated with prematurity.

CAUSES

In most cases the cause of placental abruption is unknown. There are a number of non-specific associations, including:

- high parity
- advanced maternal age
- tobacco smoking
- cocaine use
- low socio-economic group

- hypertensive disorders
- multiple pregnancy
- sudden decompression of an overdistended uterus, such as follows rupture of the membranes with polyhydramnios or after delivery of the first twin
- prolonged prelabour rupture of the membranes
- oligohydramnios
- circumvallate placenta
- trauma, such as a fall, car accident or amniocentesis (uncommon cause)
- thrombophilias (inconsistent association).

TYPES

- Revealed haemorrhage occurs when the edge of the placenta separates so there is little resistance to the blood tracking down between the membranes and the uterine wall to pass through the cervix.
- Concealed haemorrhage is much less frequent and occurs when the blood is trapped between the placenta and uterine wall and does not appear externally.
- Mixed haemorrhage occurs when there is a degree of both revealed and concealed haemorrhage (Figure 18.3).

In addition to the above classification, and depending on the amount of blood loss and the severity of the signs and symptoms, cases may be defined as mild, moderate or severe.

PATHOPHYSIOLOGY AND CLINICAL FEATURES

Haemorrhage occurs into the decidua basalis. If this bleeding is at the periphery of the placenta, the blood will track down with minimal resistance between the membranes and uterine wall and be revealed. Because there is little extravasation of blood into the myometrium, there may be minimal pain or uterine irritability and tenderness. Thus, these mild revealed cases may clinically mimic placenta praevia.

At the other extreme, the bleeding may be located more centrally and be concealed; there is retroplacental haematoma formation and, as the blood is under pressure, it may extravasate to varying degrees into the myometrium. This will increase the uterine tone, irritability and pain, probably as a result of prostaglandin release from the damaged decidual tissue. Labour often ensues. If the blood dissects through the

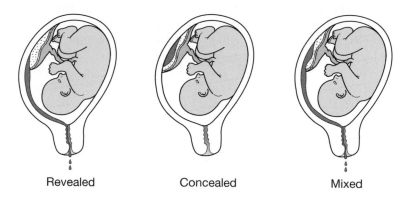

Revealed   Concealed   Mixed

Figure 18.3 Types of placental abruption

myometrium to the subserosal surface of the uterus, this discoloration can be seen at the time of caesarean section and is known as Couvelaire uterus. In the severe concealed case, there is unremitting abdominal pain and the uterus is hard and tender. The fetus dies. Decidual thromboplastins may be forced into the maternal circulation and initiate disseminated intravascular coagulation. Together with hypovolaemic shock, there is intense vasoconstriction; if this causes prolonged renal arteriolar spasm, it may lead to tubular and cortical necrosis and, ultimately, renal failure.

In between these two extreme clinical pictures, cases of mixed haemorrhage will occur.

The clinical hallmarks of placental abruption are abdominal pain, increased uterine tone and tenderness, hypovolaemic shock out of proportion to the apparent blood loss and, in more severe cases, fetal death. Ultrasound is unreliable in the diagnosis of placental abruption; it may show a retroplacental haematoma and confirm the diagnosis, but a negative ultrasound does not rule out abruption.

MANAGEMENT

Undertransfusion is a common error in cases of placental abruption. Thus, if the diagnosis of placental abruption is established, two intravenous lines should be set up and crystalloid rapidly infused. At least four units of blood should be cross-matched. In moderate and severe cases, blood transfusion will be required. A working guide to transfusion requirements is the 'rule of 30s': the recumbent pregnant woman can lose up to 30% of her blood volume and maintain a normal pulse and blood pressure; keep the haematocrit above 30% and the urinary output greater than 30 ml per hour. In severe cases, central venous pressure monitoring, if available, will guide transfusion. The management of disseminated intravascular coagulation is outlined in chapter 22.

Obstetric management will vary with the type and severity of placental abruption.[21] In mild revealed cases with no uterine tenderness, expectant treatment may be followed until 37–40 weeks of gestation, when induction of labour is undertaken based on the timing and amount of blood loss.

If the diagnosis of placental abruption is certain and the fetus is mature and alive, steps should be taken to expedite delivery. It is not uncommon for women to already be in labour when the diagnosis is established. If so, amniotomy is advisable as this will reduce the intrauterine pressure and, at least theoretically, reduce the risk of extravasation of blood and thromboplastins into the myometrium and maternal circulation. If the fetus is already dead, the labour usually progresses rapidly to spontaneous delivery. If the progress of labour is inadequate, oxytocin augmentation is appropriate. If the fetus is alive and the clinical signs are mild, the fetal heart may be monitored to anticipate vaginal delivery.

Caesarean section is used liberally for moderate and severe cases when the fetus is mature and alive, in cases unfavourable for induction of labour, if there is significant bleeding and in women in whom there is poor progress of labour after 6–8 hours.

Unclassified antepartum haemorrhage

In about 50% of cases of antepartum haemorrhage, the diagnosis of placenta praevia or placental abruption cannot be established, even after delivery. Such cases are therefore called unclassified or of unknown origin. Some of these cases are minor degrees of placenta praevia and placental abruption that cannot be confirmed. Others are probably a result of disruption of small vessels in the cervix during formation of the lower uterine segment. These are usually cases of mild bleeding that are treated expectantly; ultrasound shows no evidence of placenta praevia and there are no clinical signs of placental abruption. After initial assessment, these women can be treated outside hospital, but fetal growth and wellbeing should be followed as perinatal loss is increased in this group as a whole. Induction of labour at or close to term should be considered.

References

1. Wing DA, Paul RH, Millar LK. Management of the symptomatic placenta previa: a randomized, controlled trial of inpatient versus outpatient expectant management. *Am J Obstet Gynecol* 1996;175:806–11.
2. Droste S, Kiel K. Expectant management of placenta previa: cost–benefit analysis of outpatient treatment. *Am J Obstet Gynecol* 1994;170:1254–7.
3. Mouer JR. Placenta previa: antepartum conservative management, inpatient versus outpatient. *Am J Obstet Gynecol* 1994;170:1683–6; discussion 1685–6.
4. Rosen DM, Peek MJ. Do women with placenta praevia without antepartum haemorrhage require hospitalisation? *Aust N Z J Obstet Gynaecol* 1994;34:130–4.
5. Love CD, Wallace EM. Pregnancies complicated by placenta praevia: what is appropriate management? *Br J Obstet Gynaecol* 1996;103:864–7.
6. Lam CM, Wong SF, Chow KM, Ho LC. Women with placenta praevia and antepartum haemorrhage have a worse outcome than those who do not bleed before delivery. *J Obstet Gynaecol* 2000;20:27–31.
7. Cho JH, Jun HS, Lee CN. Hemostatic suturing technique for uterine bleeding during cesarean delivery. *Obstet Gynecol* 2000;96:129–31.
8. Lurie S, Appleman Z, Katz Z. Intractable postpartum bleeding due to placenta accreta: local vasopressin may save the uterus. *Br J Obstet Gynaecol* 1996;103:1164.
9. Quijano F, Sarmiento A, Rueda R, Caceres R. Use of Monsel's solution for placenta accreta. *Obstet Gynecol* 2008;111 Suppl:92s.
10. Bakri YN, Amri A, Abdul Jabbar F. Tamponade-balloon for obstetrical bleeding. *Int J Gynaecol Obstet* 2001;74:139–42.
11. Hansch E, Chitkara U, McAlpine J, El-Sayed Y, Dake MD, Razavi MK. Pelvic artery embolization for control of obstetric hemorrhage: a five-year experience. *Am J Obstet Gynecol* 1999;180:1454–9.
12. Baskett TF. Of violent floodings in pregnancy: evolution of the management of placenta praevia. In: Sturdee D, Oláh K, Keane D, editors. *The Yearbook of Obstetrics and Gynaecology*. Volume 9. London: RCOG Press; 2001. p. 1–14.
13. Bhide A, Thilaganathan B. Recent advances in the management of placenta previa. *Curr Opin Obstet Gynecol* 2004;16:447–51.
14. Royal College of Obstetricians and Gynaecologists. *Placenta praevia, placenta praevia accreta and vasa praevia: diagnosis and management*. Green-top Guideline No. 27. London: RCOG; 2011 [http://www.rcog.org.uk/womens-health/clinical-guidance/placenta-praevia-and-placenta-praevia-accreta-diagnosis-and-manageme].
15. ACOG Committee on Obstetric Practice. ACOG Committee opinion. Number 266, January 2002: Placenta accreta. *Obstet Gynecol* 2002;99:169–70.
16. Oyelese Y, Smulian JC. Placenta previa, placenta accreta, and vasa previa. *Obstet Gynecol* 2006;107:927–41.

17. Shrivastava V, Nageotte M, Major C, Haydon M, Wing D. Case–control comparison of cesarean hysterectomy with and without prophylactic placement of intravascular balloon catheters for placenta accreta. *Am J Obstet Gynecol* 2007;197:402e1–5.

18. Oppenheimer L; Society of Obstetricians and Gynaecologists of Canada. Diagnosis and management of placenta previa. *J Obstet Gynaecol Can* 2007;29:261–73.

19. Palacios-Jaraquemada JM. Diagnosis and management of placenta accreta. *Best Pract Res Clin Obstet Gynaecol* 2008;22:1133–48.

20. Faranesh R, Romano S, Shalev E, Salim R. Suggested approach for management of placenta percreta invading the urinary bladder. *Obstet Gynecol* 2007;110:512–15.

21. Oyelese Y, Ananth CV. Placental abruption. *Obstet Gynecol* 2006;108:1005–16.

19 Postpartum haemorrhage

Worldwide, obstetric haemorrhage is the leading cause of maternal death, such that every 2–3 minutes a woman bleeds to death in childbirth. The vast majority of these deaths are in the developing world. While haemorrhage is not the main cause of maternal mortality in the developed world, it is the largest contributor to severe maternal morbidity. Furthermore, there are reports from Australia and Canada showing an increased prevalence of severe postpartum haemorrhage (PPH).[1,2]

PPH is defined as bleeding from the genital tract in excess of 500 ml within 24 hours of vaginal delivery and in excess of 1000 ml within 24 hours of caesarean section. The reported incidence varies from 2% to 10% because blood loss is such a subjective appraisal. It is a clinical truism that doctors underestimate blood loss while patients overestimate it. This is supported by blood volume studies which show that the normal parturient loses about 500 ml of blood at vaginal delivery and 1000 ml at caesarean section. Thus, when the doctor estimates that a woman has lost 500 ml at vaginal delivery, she has probably lost closer to 1 litre. Therefore, in terms of clinical management, the working definition of an estimated 500 ml blood loss is a reasonable one. It is also advisable to have a lower tolerance for blood loss with small women who have a smaller blood volume and in those who are already anaemic. Because of the latter two factors, some define PPH as over 500 ml estimated blood loss or that which causes haemodynamic changes.

Aetiology

UTERINE ATONY

Uterine atony is the cause of PPH in 80–85% of cases. Uterine atony is attributable to a failure of or interference with the normal mechanisms that ensure the haemostatic contraction and retraction of the uterine musculature (see chapter 5). It can occur in normal labour but is more often associated with:

- high parity
- overdistention of the uterus with multiple pregnancy, poly-hydramnios and fetal macrosomia
- prolonged, precipitate or induced labour
- antepartum haemorrhage: both placenta praevia and placental abruption
- drugs: tocolytic agents and general anaesthesia with fluorinated hydrocarbons
- retained placenta, placental fragments and blood clots (see chapter 5)
- structural abnormalities of the uterus, such as uterine fibroids or anomalies, as these may interfere with uterine retraction
- mismanagement of the third stage with manipulation of the fundus and premature cord traction as this can lead to partial separation of the placenta and increased blood loss.

GENITAL TRACT TRAUMA

Genital tract trauma is the second most common cause of PPH, accounting for 10–15% of cases:

- episiotomy
- lacerations of the perineum, vagina and cervix
- laceration or rupture of the uterus
- vulvovaginal and broad ligament haematomas.

Acute uterine inversion and disseminated intravascular coagulation are additional but uncommon causes of PPH (see chapters 20 and 22).

Medical management

PREVENTION

The prevention of PPH by active management of the third stage of labour is discussed in chapter 5.

UTERINE MASSAGE

The first step in the management of atonic postpartum haemorrhage is to contract the uterus. The first thing to hand is, in fact, the hand, which should be used to apply firm but gentle fundal massage.

OXYTOCIC DRUGS

Oxytocic drugs are covered in detail in chapter 5, but their specific application in the management of uterine atony is as follows:

- Give oxytocin five units intravenously. This can be repeated within a few minutes if required.

- Give 40 units of oxytocin in 500 ml crystalloid solution run in briskly to initiate and continue uterine contraction.

Although oxytocin will control most cases of atonic PPH, it is not uncommon for the myometrial oxytocin receptors to be downregulated and unresponsive, particularly after many hours of induction or augmentation with oxytocin. Thus, if the uterus does not contract promptly after giving oxytocin, do not hesitate to move on to ergometrine and/or the prostaglandins:

- Give ergometrine 0.2 mg by intravenous injection over 2 minutes or 0.25 mg by the intramuscular route (if not contraindicated).

- Misoprostol is increasingly being chosen as the uterotonic of second choice. It can be given as 400–600 micrograms sublingually or 800–1000 micrograms rectally.

- 15-methyl prostaglandin F2α 0.25 mg is given by intramuscular or intramyometrial injection. It can also be administered as a dilute infusion of 0.25 mg in 500 ml saline.

In general, oxytocic drugs are more likely to fail in cases of prolonged labour with chorioamnionitis, where the exhausted and infected myometrium does not contract well.

On rare occasions, the uterus that is unresponsive to oxytocic drugs will contract with continuous uterine massage. This should be vigorous but not so hard as to cause pain to the woman. In cases with persistent ooze, the woman can be taught to massage her own uterine fundus.

TREAT HYPOVOLAEMIA

With postpartum haemorrhage there should be early recourse to rapid intravenous infusion of crystalloid (Ringer's lactate or normal saline).

- Two intravenous lines of access should be established with 14–16-gauge cannulas (intravenous crystalloid can be infused twice as fast through a 14-gauge cannula compared with an 18-gauge cannula).

- In healthy, non-anaemic women, blood loss of up to 1500 ml can usually be managed with rapid infusion of crystalloid. This assumes that the bleeding has been arrested. In the woman who is already anaemic, or in the woman with blood loss of 2000 ml or more, transfusion of packed red cells will be necessary.

- If the blood loss is massive and the woman has hypovolaemic shock, both intravenous crystalloid and colloid, in the form of 5% albumin or plasmanate, will be required until blood is available. As albumin is very viscous, it should be drawn up with a wide-bore needle and added to saline so that it can be rapidly infused. Some of the principles of transfusion are outlined in chapter 22.

BIMANUAL UTERINE COMPRESSION

The vaginal hand formed as a fist in the anterior fornix and the abdominal hand cupping and pushing down on the posterofundal part of the uterus may provide temporary compression and reduction of bleeding (Figure 19.1). In addition, rotary massage between the fist and hand may help contract the uterus. This is painful and can be used only in the short term or in women receiving epidural analgesia. Bimanual uterine compression is used as a temporary measure before moving to surgical options.

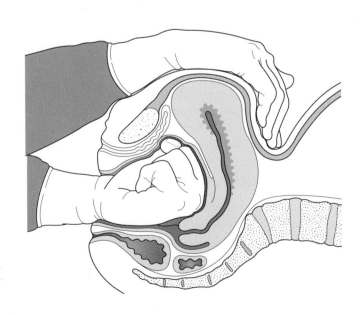

Figure 19.1 Bimanual compression of the uterus

AORTIC COMPRESSION

Aortic compression is a fairly desperate move that may be tried in the thin woman. One hand pulls the uterine fundus out of the pelvis and pushes upwards and backwards across the lower part of the uterus, while the other hand directs the fundus posteriorly to compress the aorta. This may be of limited value if the uterine fundus is atonic and too soft to provide an adequate compression pad. Alternatively, the fist can be used just above the umbilicus with the heel of the hand pressing down on the aorta. Aortic compression is used as a temporary measure before moving to surgical options.

ANTI-SHOCK GARMENT

In some areas, when delay in transfer and/or the availability of surgical management is anticipated, the use of the anti-shock garment may be life-saving.[3]

Surgical management

The management of lacerations and haematomas of the lower genital tract is covered in chapter 6. There are a number of surgical approaches that may be applicable for uterine haemorrhage. Depending upon the circumstances, these may include the following.[4]

UTERINE TAMPONADE

Since the early 1990s, uterine tamponade, which had largely fallen out of favour, has re-emerged as a potentially uterus-saving technique.[5] There are two approaches. One is the more traditional tight packing of the uterus with a 10 cm wide gauze roll; this requires general or regional anaesthesia and the success or failure is not known until the bleeding does or does not seep through the pack. Some will use a plastic bag placed in the uterus to facilitate complete packing of the uterine cavity and also to ease its removal after 12–24 hours. The other approach is to use a balloon device for tamponade. This was first carried out by adopting available balloons such as the Sengstaken–Blakemore tube or the Rüsch urological balloon. A custom-designed balloon has been devised for this purpose, which in essence is like a large Foley catheter: the Bakri balloon.[6] Others have improvised and used a condom or a surgical glove tied to a straight plastic urinary catheter.

The balloon is placed in the uterine cavity, a process that does not require full anaesthesia, and filled with fluid using a large syringe. Once the balloon is seen to be bulging at the cervix, it is adequately filled; this usually requires 250–350 ml of fluid, but in some cases up to 500 ml is needed. One can then observe whether the bleeding has stopped, which is usually apparent within a few minutes: the so-called 'tamponade' test.[7] If successful, the vagina is then packed with 10 cm gauze roll and a Foley catheter placed in the bladder. The catheter is kept in place for 12–24 hours and then gradually deflated over several hours and removed. Intrauterine tamponade is best covered with prophylactic antibiotics and continuous infusion of oxytocin to promote uterine contractions.

MAJOR VESSEL EMBOLISATION

Angiographic embolisation of branches of the internal iliac artery has been used successfully to control haemorrhage from uterine atony as well as trauma to the cervix, paracolpos and upper vagina.[8] Some of the surgical measures mentioned above may be only partially successful but should sustain the woman until embolisation can be organised. Embolisation can be performed under local anaesthesia together with mild sedation. Under angiographic control, and through a femoral artery puncture, a catheter is guided to the aortic bifurcation and then in turn to each of the internal iliac arteries and their branches. Bleeding vessels are identified by extravasation of contrast material and blocked by the injection of gelatin particles.

MAJOR VESSEL LIGATION

If the abdomen is open and one is dealing directly with haemorrhage following caesarean section or uterine rupture, major vessel ligation may be indicated. The most logical approach for uterine haemorrhage is a combination of uterine artery and ovarian artery ligation. Luckily, this is very simple and can be performed rapidly by any general obstetrician (Figure 19.2).[9,10] The placement of the suture, which ligates the ascending branch of the uterine artery, is approximately 2 cm below the level of a transverse lower-segment caesarean section incision. Using a large curved needle and a No. 1 absorbable suture, pass the needle through the myometrium from front to back about 2 cm in from the side of the uterus. Transilluminate the broad ligament and bring the needle back through an avascular portion to encircle the uterine vessels. Tie the suture firmly to compress the uterine vessels; this is facilitated and stabilised by the portion of myometrium included in the stitch. Before passing the suture, ensure that the bladder is well down to avoid injury to the lower urinary tract. Repeat the procedure on the opposite side.

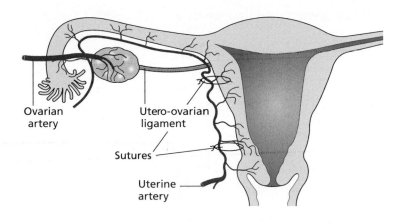

Ovarian
artery

Utero-ovarian
ligament

Sutures

Uterine
artery

Figure 19.2 Uterine and ovarian artery ligation

Branches of the ovarian artery pass above the ovary and then down to anastomose with the branches of the ascending uterine artery below the uterine attachment of the utero-ovarian ligament. Place an encircling suture just below the utero-ovarian ligament in an identical manner to that used for the uterine artery below. Repeat on the other side. Ligating the ovarian artery at this point does not interfere with the blood supply to the ovary or tube. The uterine arteries usually recanalise and subsequent menstrual and reproductive function is normal. Bilateral uterine and ovarian artery ligation can be achieved swiftly and safely and is often effective in dealing with uterine haemorrhage attributable to trauma or atony.

Internal iliac artery ligation may be considered for haemorrhage from the cervix, paracolpos and upper vagina.[11] Unless the abdomen is already open, it is better to approach these lacerations with direct suture by the vaginal route and, if this fails, move to major vessel embolisation. However, if the abdomen is already open, or if facilities for vessel embolisation are not available, it is logical to try and deal with the haemorrhage directly. The descending branch of the uterine artery supplies the cervix, vagina and paracolpos. Thus, haemorrhage from these areas is more logically approached by internal iliac artery ligation.

The technique is as follows: raise the mid-portion of the round ligament with a Babcock clamp and enter the retroperitoneal space between this portion of the round ligament and the fallopian tube. With a finger, suction tip or a moist sponge stick, the space is easily opened to the pelvic side wall. The bifurcation of the common iliac artery can be seen or palpated. The ureter and its attached peritoneum is adjacent to

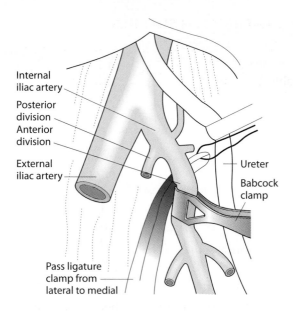

Figure 19.3 Internal iliac artery ligation

this bifurcation and must be identified and reflected medially (Figure 19.3). The external iliac artery passes laterally and superiorly, with the internal iliac artery passing downwards and medially. Gently clear the areola tissue from the first 3 cm of the internal iliac branch. The artery can then be elevated very gently with a Babcock clamp and a right angle clamp containing a doubled absorbable No. 1 suture passed from lateral to medial beneath the artery. This should be done between 2 cm and 3 cm from the origin of the internal iliac artery. Great care must be taken not to damage the adjacent veins underneath the artery. The artery is then doubly ligated but not divided.

Owing to the presence of major collateral anastomoses in the pelvis between the lumbar and iliolumbar arteries, the middle sacral and lateral sacral arteries and the superior and middle haemorrhoidal arteries, the effectiveness of internal iliac artery ligation is limited. This technique has been shown to reduce the pulse pressure within the arterial system by about 85% and, in essence, reduces it to that of a venous system, thereby giving the normal clotting system a chance to work.[12] However, it is only about 50% effective in controlling haemorrhage in which medical management and uterine artery ligation have failed.[13,14] Another drawback is that, with ligation of the internal iliac artery, access for subsequent angiographic embolisation of vessels is restricted.

UTERINE COMPRESSION SUTURES

Improvised uterine compression sutures, such as large figure-of-eight sutures across the lower uterine segment in cases of placenta praevia, have probably been in use since the beginning of the 20th century. However, the first standardised technique was described in 1997 by B-Lynch, who named the technique after himself.[15] There have been a number of modifications since then and the main ones are described below.

B-Lynch suture

The main role of the B-Lynch suture technique is in the management of uterine atony that is refractory to uterotonic drugs at the time of caesarean section. With the patient in the Lloyd-Davis (froglegged) position, an assistant clears out any vaginal clots and observes the effect of manual uterine compression by the operator. If this manual compression stops the bleeding, the compression suture should be effective.

Using a large (≥70 mm) round-bodied needle, the suture is first passed into the uterine cavity 3 cm below the transverse caesarean incision and about 4 cm in from the lateral wall of the uterus. This suture exits the uterus at a similar point above the incision and is looped over the uterine fundus to the back of the uterus opposite the caesarean incision. At this point, the suture is again passed into the uterine cavity and across the inner back wall to a similar point on the other side where the needle exits the uterus. The suture is then looped back over the uterine fundus and down the anterior surface to enter above and exit below the margins of the transverse incision to mirror the placement on the other side (Figure 19.4). The uterine incision is closed with a separate suture. While the assistant manually compresses the uterus, the suture is

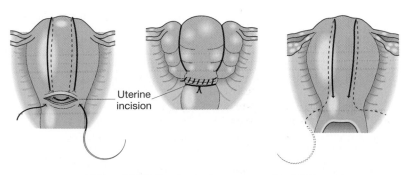

Uterine incision

Figure 19.4 B-Lynch uterine compression suture

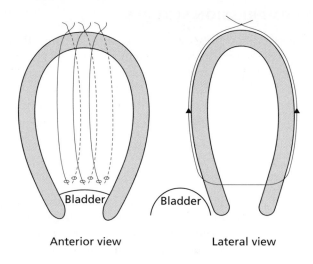

Anterior view   Lateral view

Figure 19.5 Vertical uterine compression suture

progressively tightened. This incremental compression and tightening of the suture is very important. The two ends are then tied below the uterine incision. A No. 1 Monocryl (Ethicon; polyglecaprone 25) suture on a 70 mm blunt semicircular needle is available for this purpose.[16]

Vertical compression suture

The vertical compression suture is a simplification of the B-Lynch suture that can be used when there is no caesarean incision.[17] Just above the bladder reflection, using a straight 10 cm needle, the absorbable suture is passed through the uterus from front to back (Figure 19.5). The suture is looped on each side to the uterine fundus and tied there. Two sutures are usually placed but quite often more are needed if the uterus is broad. To avoid any tendency of the sutures to slide down off the sides of the uterus, the sutures should be tied together at the fundus.

Square compression sutures

Square compression sutures involve the direct apposition of the anterior and posterior walls of the uterus by passing a straight needle back and forth in a square configuration with about 3 cm spacing[18] (Figure 19.6).

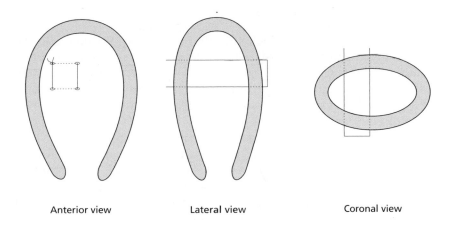

| Anterior view | Lateral view | Coronal view |

Figure 19.6 Square uterine compression suture

In this way the anterior and posterior walls are compressed together as the suture is tied down. This can be repeated at several sites and, if necessary, can cover the whole uterus. Square compression sutures have a special application in cases of placenta praevia bleeding from the lower uterine segment, with or without areas of accreta (see chapter 18, page 200).

Rare complications of compression sutures include pyometra and ischaemic necrosis.[19,20] Experience with subsequent fertility and pregnancy outcome is limited but reassuring.[21] The above compression suture techniques represent a simple alternative to hysterectomy and are 80–90% successful in stopping haemorrhage and saving the uterus.[21]

HYSTERECTOMY

The aim of all of the above measures is to try and preserve the uterus. However, there comes a time in the face of continued and unrelenting haemorrhage when one has to accept the failure of other measures and move to hysterectomy. This requires a fine clinical balance between the systematic application of conservative surgical measures and excessive delay, potentially leading to increasing transfusion requirements and the development of disseminated intravascular coagulation. The decision will be influenced by the woman's age, parity and desire for future children. The technical aspects of obstetric hysterectomy are covered in chapter 16.

PREPAREDNESS FOR PPH

Cases of severe PPH in which the above surgical measures may be required are relatively rare, and the equipment necessary is often not in common use or readily to hand. Valuable time can be lost while staff who are unfamiliar with the required materials and their whereabouts on the labour unit seek the necessary equipment. Given that severe PPH is predictably unpredictable, it is wise to have a PPH bundle or tray placed prominently beside the obstetric operating theatre which contains the necessary items:[22] appropriate sutures and needles for major vessel ligation and compression sutures, uterine packing and a balloon device for uterine tamponade, vaginal retractors for exposure of cervical and high vaginal lacerations and diagrams to aid the placement of uterine compression and major vessel ligation sutures. Education, audit and simulation drills by labour ward staff may help reduce delay and guide logical management in cases of severe PPH.[23–25] The sequence of steps, from simple to complex, has been described in algorithm form and endorsed in guidelines.[26,27]

References

1. Cameron CA, Roberts CL, Olive EC, Ford JB, Fischer WE. Trends in postpartum haemorrhage. *Aust N Z J Public Health* 2006;30:151–6.
2. Joseph KS, Rouleau J, Kramer MS, Young DC, Liston RM, Baskett TF; Maternal Health Study Group of the Canadian Perinatal Surveillance System. Investigation of an increase in postpartum haemorrhage in Canada. *BJOG* 2007;114:751–9.
3. Miller S, Martin HB, Morris JL. Anti-shock garment in postpartum haemorrhage. *Best Pract Res Clin Obstet Gynaecol* 2008;22:1057–74.
4. Chandraharan E, Arulkumaran S. Surgical aspects of postpartum haemorrhage. *Best Pract Res Clin Obstet Gynaecol* 2008;22:1089–102.
5. Maier RC. Control of postpartum hemorrhage with uterine packing. *Am J Obstet Gynecol* 1993;169:317-21; discussion 321–3.
6. Bakri YN, Amir A, Abdul Jabbar F. Tamponade-balloon for obstetrical bleeding. *Int J Gynecol Obstet* 2001;74:139–42.
7. Condous GS, Arulkumaran S, Symonds I, Chapman R, Sinha A, Razvi K. The "tamponade test" in the management of massive postpartum hemorrhage. *Obstet Gynecol* 2003;101:767–72.
8. Lee JS, Shepherd SM. Endovascular treatment of postpartum hemorrhage. *Clin Obstet Gynecol* 2010;53:209–18.
9. Fahmy K. Uterine artery ligation to control postpartum haemorrhage. *Int J Gynaecol Obstet* 1987;25:363–7.
10. AbdRabbo SA. Stepwise uterine devascularization: a novel technique for management of uncontrolled postpartum hemorrhage with preservation of the uterus. *Am J Obstet Gynecol* 1994;171;694–700.

11. Clark SL, Phelan JP, Yeh SY, Bruce SR, Paul RH. Hypogastric artery ligation for obstetric hemorrhage. *Obstet Gynecol* 1985;66:353–6.
12. Burchell RC. Physiology of internal iliac artery ligation. *J Obstet Gynaecol Br Commonw* 1968;75:642–51.
13. Evans S, McShane P. The efficacy of internal iliac ligation in obstetric hemorrhage. *Surg Gynecol Obstet* 1985;162:250–3.
14. Joshi VM, Otiv SR, Majunder R, Nikam YA, Shrivastava M. Internal iliac artery ligation for arresting postpartum haemorrhage. *BJOG* 2007;114:356–61.
15. B-Lynch C, Coker A, Lawal AH, Abu J, Cowan MJ. The B-Lynch surgical technique for the control of massive postpartum haemorrhage: an alternative to hysterectomy? Five cases reported. *Br J Obstet Gynaecol* 1997;104:372–5.
16. Price N, B-Lynch C. Technical description of the B-Lynch brace suture for treatment of massive postpartum haemorrhage and review of published cases. *Int J Fertil Womens Med* 2005;50:148–63.
17. Hayman RC, Arulkumaran S, Steer PJ. Uterine compression sutures: surgical management of postpartum hemorrhage. *Obstet Gynecol* 2002;99:502–6.
18. Cho JH, Jun HS, Lee CN. Hemostatic suturing technique for uterine bleeding during cesarean delivery. *Obstet Gynecol* 2000;96:129–31.
19. Ochoa M, Allaire AD, Stitely ML. Pyometria after hemostatic square suture technique. *Obstet Gynecol* 2002;99:506–9.
20. Treloar EJ, Anderson RS, Andrews HS, Bailey JL. Uterine necrosis following B-Lynch suture for primary postpartum haemorrhage. *BJOG* 2006;113:486–8.
21. Baskett TF. Uterine compression sutures for postpartum hemorrhage: efficacy, morbidity, and subsequent pregnancy. *Obstet Gynecol* 2007;110:68–71.
22. Baskett TF. Surgical management of severe obstetric haemorrhage: experience with an obstetric haemorrhage equipment tray. *J Obstet Gynaecol Can* 2004;26:805–8.
23. Rizvi F, Mackey R, Barrett T, McKenna P, Geary M. Successful reduction of massive postpartum haemorrhage by use of guidelines and staff education. *BJOG* 2004;111:495–8.
24. Clark EA, Fisher J, Arafeh J, Druzin M. Team training/simulation. *Clin Obstet Gynecol* 2010;53:265–77.
25. Skupski DW, Lowenwirt IP, Weinbaum FI, Brodsky D, Danek M, Eglinton GS. Improving hospital systems for the care of women with major obstetric hemorrhage. *Obstet Gynecol* 2006;107:977–83.
26. Chandraharan E, Arulkumaran S. Management algorithm for atonic postpartum haemorrhage. *J Paediatr Obstet Gynaecol* 2005;12:106–12.
27. Royal College of Obstetricians and Gynaecologists. *Prevention and management of postpartum haemorrhage*. Green-top Guideline No. 52. London: RCOG; 2009 [http://www.rcog.org.uk/womens-health/clinical-guidance/prevention-and-management-postpartum-haemorrhage-green-top-52].

20 Acute uterine inversion

The frequency of acute uterine inversion, a rare but life-threatening condition, depends upon the standard of care during the third stage of labour. The incidence therefore varies widely from about 1/2000 to 1/50 000 deliveries.

The degree of inversion may be incomplete, in which the fundus is inverted but does not protrude through the cervix (first degree), or complete, when the inverted fundus passes completely through the cervix and lies either in the vagina (second degree) or completely outside the introitus (third degree) (Figure 20.1).

Causes

The combination of uterine relaxation and fundal insertion of the placenta provides the important predisposition to acute uterine inversion, a predisposition which may then be converted to uterine inversion by the factors discussed below.[1]

- Mismanagement of the third stage of labour is the cause in the majority of cases, either by pressure on the uterine fundus or by premature traction on the umbilical cord before the placenta has separated and when the uterus is relaxed. This provides additional support in favour of active management of the third stage of labour, because the administered oxytocic and ensuing uterine contraction make it impossible to turn the uterus inside out.

- An acute rise in intra-abdominal pressure as a result of maternal coughing or vomiting can rarely produce a strong enough propulsive force on the uterine fundus to cause inversion, if the vulnerable set-up of a fundally implanted placenta and uterine relaxation are present.

- Manual removal of the placenta, if performed rapidly and a portion of the placenta remains attached to the uterine wall, can lead to acute uterine inversion. This can also occur with those who routinely, albeit inadvisably, carry out routine manual removal of the placenta before the uterus has contracted at the time of caesarean section.

- Rare causes include an abnormally short cord or a connective tissue disorder such as Marfan's syndrome.[2]

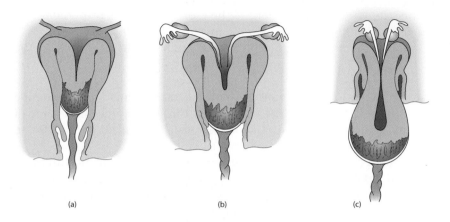

(a)   (b)   (c)

Figure 20.1 Degrees of uterine inversion: (a) first degree (incomplete); (b) second degree (complete – within the vagina); (c) third degree (complete – outside the introitus)

Clinical features

- The diagnosis of acute uterine inversion may be obvious, with the sudden appearance of a boggy mass in the vagina or at the introitus.
- Persistent hypogastric pain and pelvic pressure during and after the third stage of labour also suggest acute uterine inversion.
- Sudden onset of shock with profound hypotension, bradycardia and pallor. Initially, the shock is of a neurogenic type with vagal inhibition owing to traction on the infundibulopelvic, round and ovarian ligaments. This is usually soon followed by hypovolaemic shock from the concurrent bleeding.[1,3,4]
- If the woman is not overweight, one may note the absence of the uterine fundus on abdominal palpation.
- Incomplete inversion can be more difficult to diagnose and usually presents with persistent bleeding. In a thin woman it may be possible to palpate the dimple in the fundus of the uterus, but incomplete inversion is usually discovered only during manual exploration of the uterus performed because of the continued bleeding.

Management

Immediately after uterine inversion, the cervical ring will constrict and cause increasing congestion of the inverted fundus. Occasionally, if immediate manual replacement of the uterine fundus is carried out, the cervical ring will be relaxed enough to allow successful reduction. Thus, if you are present when acute inversion occurs, immediately cup the uterine fundus in the palm of your hand, replace it in the vagina and push upwards towards the umbilicus. If the cervical ring is still relaxed, this may allow successful replacement. Usually, however, this is not the case and preparations should be made for resuscitation, anaesthesia and manual replacement of the uterus, as detailed below.

- First, summon assistance in the form of nursing and anaesthesia personnel.

- Pre-empt and/or correct the inevitable hypovolaemia that follows the initial neurogenic shock. Two intravenous lines should be established with wide-bore cannulas and crystalloid should be rapidly infused. Four units of blood should be cross-matched. Place a Foley catheter in the bladder. Even in hospitals with readily available anaesthesia, a significant proportion of these cases require transfusion.[1,3]

- If the uterus has descended through the introitus, replace it in the vagina and raise the end of the bed to decrease the stretch, and therefore the parasympathetic stimulus on the infundibulo pelvic ligaments.

- If regional anaesthesia (spinal or epidural) is in place, it may only be necessary to add a tocolytic for uterine relaxation to allow manual replacement.[5] This is usually best achieved with glyceryl trinitrate; the details of glyceryl trinitrate administration are covered in chapter 23, page 246. If there is no regional anaesthesia in place, general anaesthesia is usually given with one of the fluorinated hydrocarbons (sevoflurane or isoflurane) to aid uterine relaxation.

- Once anaesthesia and uterine relaxation have been achieved, manual replacement of the uterus is undertaken. If the placenta is still completely attached, do not remove it as this will increase blood loss. If the placenta is only partially attached, remove the attached portion before manual replacement.

- The portion of the uterus that came down first (the uterine fundus) is replaced last. Thus, cup the fundus in the palm of the hand and, with the extended fingers and thumb, press on the lower uterine segment as it protrudes through the cervical ring. With pressure from the palm of the hand and the fingers, the lower segment and adjacent portion of the upper uterine segment should be squeezed through the

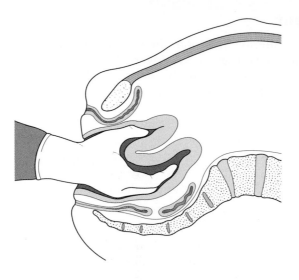

Figure 20.2 Manual replacement of inverted uterus

constricting ring followed by the uterine fundus (Figure 20.2). Care should be taken not to forcibly manipulate the lower uterine segment, which may be thin and prone to tearing. Manual replacement may take sustained effort for up to 3–5 minutes. Once the inversion has been corrected and the placenta, if still attached, has been removed, the hand should be withdrawn and an oxytocin infusion run to contract the uterus. The uterus is re-explored to make sure it is intact and there are no remaining placental fragments. The vaginal fornices should also be carefully inspected for lacerations. The oxytocin infusion should be continued for 8–12 hours. Provided anaesthesia is available within 2 hours of the event, manual replacement of the uterus is usually successful.

- In cases in which manual replacement is unsuccessful, the hydrostatic method described by O'Sullivan can be used.[6,7] The principle of this method is to distend the vaginal fornices with fluid, which pulls outwards on the constricting cervical ring and also applies pressure on the fundus, thereby allowing replacement of the inversion. Having ensured that there are no tears in the vagina, cervix or uterus, intravenous tubing is guided into the posterior fornix while the other hand seals the vulva around the wrist. Warm saline is then fed through the tubing using a pressure infuser: 3–5 litres may be required (Figure 20.3). A variation on this technique is to attach the

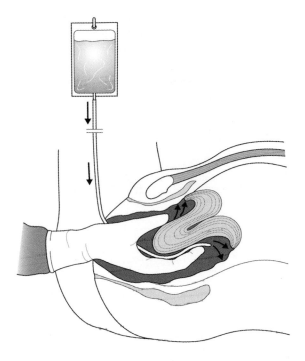

Figure 20.3 Hydrostatic method of replacing inverted uterus

tubing to a silastic vacuum extractor cup, which can be placed inside the introitus to provide a better seal and prevent egress of the fluid.[8] In cases of failed manual replacement, the hydrostatic method can be both atraumatic and comfortingly effective.

- In exceptional cases of neglected uterine inversion, the above treatments may not succeed. On these rare occasions, laparotomy is required to effect Huntington's operation, which involves sequential traction on the inverted fundus with tenacula until the fundus is reduced.[9] It may be possible at laparotomy to replace the uterine fundus without tenacula by placing the hands at the front and back of the uterus, such that the fingers extend below the inverted fundus at the level of the lower uterine segment. Persistent and progressive pressure from the flexed fingertips may allow restoration of the uterine fundus without the use of tenacula. Others have suggested a soft silastic vacuum cup be placed in the crater and the fundus 'extracted' to its correct position.[10] Occasionally, at laparotomy the constriction ring is too tight to allow Huntington's technique, in

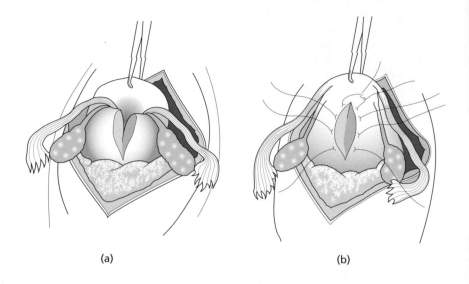

(a)   (b)

Figure 20.4 Haultain's operation: (a) incision of posterior constriction ring; (b) suture of incision after replacement

which case Haultain's operation is used with incision of the cervical constriction ring posteriorly.[11] This allows correction of the inversion; the incised portion of the lower uterus is then sutured (Figure 20.4).

- A broad-spectrum antibiotic should be given for 24–48 hours post-partum.

If acute uterine inversion occurs in circumstances without available anaesthesia, replacement can sometimes be achieved with a combination of intravenous narcotic, inhalation analgesia, combined pudendal and paracervical block and a tocolytic drug such as glyceryl trinitrate. In these circumstances, if a gentle attempt at manual replacement is unsuccessful, O'Sullivan's hydrostatic method should be used.

It bears re-emphasis that the majority of these life-threatening cases are associated with mismanagement of the third stage of labour and are, therefore, preventable.

References

1. Baskett TF. Acute uterine inversion: a review of 40 cases. *J Obstet Gynaecol Can* 2002;24:953–6.
2. Quinn RJ, Mukerjee B. Spontaneous uterine inversion in association with Marfan's syndrome. *Aust N Z J Obstet Gynaecol* 1982;22:163–4.

3. Dickson MJ, Anders NK. Acute puerperal uterine inversion: a report of five cases. *J Obstet Gynaecol* 2000;20:426–7.
4. Achanna S, Mohamed Z, Krishnan M. Puerperal uterine inversion: a report of four cases. *J Obstet Gynaecol Res* 2006;32:341–5.
5. Brar HS, Greenspoon JS, Platt LD, Paul RH. Acute puerperal uterine inversion. New approaches to management. *J Reprod Med* 1989;34:173–7.
6. O'Sullivan JV. Acute inversion of the uterus. *Br Med J* 1945;2:282–3.
7. Momani AW, Hassan A. Treatment of puerperal uterine inversion by the hydrostatic method; reports of five cases. *Eur J Obstet Gynecol Reprod Biol* 1989;32:281–5.
8. Ogueh O, Ayida G. Acute uterine inversion: a new technique of hydrostatic replacement. *Br J Obstet Gynaecol* 1997;104:951–2.
9. Huntington JL. Acute inversion of the uterus. *Boston Med Surg J* 1921;184:376–80.
10. Antonelli E, Irion O, Tolck P, Morales M. Subacute uterine inversion: description of a novel replacement technique using the obstetric ventouse. *BJOG* 2006;113:846–7.
11. Haultain FWN. The treatment of chronic uterine inversion by abdominal hysterectomy, with a successful case. *Br Med J* 1901;2:974.

21 Amniotic fluid embolism

Although a rare event, occurring in 1/25 000–80 000 deliveries, amniotic fluid embolism (AFE) is perhaps the most catastrophic of all obstetric complications. In the developed world, AFE accounts for approximately 10% of all direct maternal deaths, rating it among the top three causes.[1-3] The prominence of AFE is accounted for by the fact that, although it is a rare condition, the mortality rate is 30–80% and, even among survivors, the hypoxic insult is so profound that many have permanent neurological damage. There is some evidence that prompt resuscitation and intensive care lead to improved intact survival.[4,5]

Pathophysiology

The pathophysiology of AFE is poorly understood. It has been suggested that many of the hallmarks of AFE are similar to those of septic shock and anaphylaxis.[6-9] Furthermore, it has been established that amniotic fluid commonly enters the maternal circulation without ill effect in most women.[10] It is postulated that in certain susceptible women, fetal cells and other vasoactive substances, such as prostaglandins and leukotrienes, may initiate, via endogenous mediators, a complex pathophysiological cascade similar to that seen in anaphylactic and septic shock. The sequelae are as follows:

- Initially, there is acute pulmonary arteriolar obstruction and hypertension. This is transient and soon followed by left ventricular failure resulting in profound hypotension.[5,11,12]

- Next, there is severe hypoxia as a result of ventilation–perfusion imbalance. This, together with the hypotension, produces a generalised hypoxia, often leading to seizures. It is this profound and sustained hypoxia that is responsible for the neurological damage in survivors.

- Disseminated intravascular coagulation (DIC) is an almost universal finding in those who survive longer than 1 hour. DIC is probably caused by fetal antigens and tissue factors in the amniotic fluid activating the coagulation cascade.[13] The DIC is almost certainly compounded by the continuing hypoxia.

Clinical features

ASSOCIATED FACTORS

Reviews have shown that there are no consistent risk factors for AFE.[2,3,5,6,14] AFE is more likely to occur in late pregnancy, but it can occur in association with first- and second-trimester miscarriage. Amniotic fluid may gain entry to the maternal circulation during spontaneous labour and delivery or at the time of amniotomy or caesarean section. There are minor associations with certain factors such as increasing maternal age, high parity, multiple pregnancy, eclampsia, placental abruption, induction or augmentation of labour, operative delivery, cervical laceration and minor procedures such as intrauterine pressure catheter insertion, amnioinfusion and amniotomy.[3,5,15,16] Some reviews suggest that uterine hyperstimulation is a potential factor which should be avoided.[17] However, these associations are quite inconsistent and the condition is therefore unpredictable. The majority of cases occur during labour or just after delivery. On rare occasions, the acute manifestations of amniotic fluid embolism may be delayed for 2–4 hours following delivery.[18]

CLINICAL PRESENTATION

Clinical signs and symptoms of AFE include most or all of the following:

- restlessness, lightheadedness, paraesthesia, nausea and vomiting
- acute respiratory distress, chest discomfort and cyanosis
- profound hypotension and cardiovascular collapse
- severe hypoxia with loss of consciousness, seizures and/or coma
- haemorrhage and DIC develop in almost all cases if the woman survives for 1–2 hours.

If the fetus has not been delivered, the maternal hypoxia will soon result in fetal hypoxia manifested by fetal heart rate abnormalities. On occasion, there may be tetanic uterine contractions soon after amniotic fluid embolism; these contractions are usually the result of the embolism rather than the cause.

DIAGNOSIS

The differential diagnosis of AFE includes other acute events such as gastric acid aspiration into the lungs, thrombotic pulmonary embolism, myocardial infarction, eclampsia and anaphylactic drug reaction. In most cases, clinical features should distinguish these conditions.

In essence, the sudden onset of cardiopulmonary collapse, together with coma or seizures, in labour at or shortly after delivery in the woman with no other apparent predisposing causes should prompt the diagnosis of AFE. Even if the diagnosis is not completely secure at this stage, the initial management of cardiorespiratory collapse attributable to any of the above causes is the same: cardiopulmonary resuscitation.

The definitive diagnosis of AFE is said to be confirmed by the presence of amniotic fluid debris in the maternal circulation. This can be demonstrated at postmortem examination in the pulmonary precapillary arterioles using special fat stains and immunohistochemical techniques to identify fetal isoantigens.[19] In survivors, blood to test for fetal squamous cells may be obtained from the right side of the heart via a central line; however, it has been shown that this situation may occur in normal pregnancy.[10] Thus, the diagnosis is now largely based on the combination of a clear clinical picture, postmortem analysis and newer immunohistochemical techniques,[20] with the presence of squames in the maternal circulation a secondary feature.

Management

The principles of management of AFE are resuscitation and intensive care:

- Cardiopulmonary resuscitation, which will include intubation and oxygenation by intermittent positive pressure ventilation.

- Circulatory support with intravenous dopamine infusion, which may help maintain adequate cardiac output. This is best guided by experts together with more sophisticated monitoring, including central venous pressure and systemic and pulmonary arterial lines.

- Although there is no proof of their value, many will use high-dose steroids such as intravenous hydrocortisone 500 mg every 6 hours.

- If the woman survives long enough, DIC will almost certainly ensue. The principles of managing this complication are outlined in chapter 22, page 241.

- Some benefit has been found from plasma exchange and haemofiltration to aid clearance and 'wash out' of the amniotic fluid and vasoactive substances from the circulation.[21]

- If the fetus has not already been delivered, steps should be taken to do so immediately: vaginally if safe and feasible and, if not, by immediate caesarean section. Not only will the fetus rapidly become hypoxic and need to be delivered, but resuscitation of the mother will be aided by delivery of the fetus.[4] Unfortunately, the incidence of neurological damage in both maternal and neonatal survivors is high in this devastating condition.

FE is so rare that most obstetricians will never encounter a case in their reer. National registries have been established in an attempt to gather enough cases to provide insight into this enigmatic and unpredictable condition.[6,22]

References

1. Lewis G (editor). The Confidential Enquiry into Maternal and Child Health (CEMACH). *Saving Mothers' Lives: Reviewing Maternal Deaths to Make Motherhood Safer 2003–2005. The Seventh Report on Confidential Enquiries into Maternal Deaths in the United Kingdom.* London: CEMACH; 2007.
2. Burrows A, Khoo SK. The amniotic fluid embolism syndrome: 10 years' experience at a major teaching hospital. *Aust N Z J Obstet Gynaecol* 1995;35:245–50.
3. Spiliopoulos M, Puri I, Jain NJ, Kruse L, Mastrogiannis D, Dandolu V. Amniotic fluid embolism – risk factors, maternal and neonatal outcomes. *J Matern Fetal Neonatal Med* 2009;22:439–44.
4. Gilbert WM, Danielson B. Amniotic fluid embolism: decreased mortality in a population-based study. *Obstet Gynecol* 1999;93:973–7.
5. Conde-Agudelo A, Romero R. Amniotic fluid embolism: an evidence-based review. *Am J Obstet Gynecol* 2009;201:445.e1–13.
6. Clark SL, Hawkins GD, Dudley DA, Dildy GA, Porter TF. Amniotic fluid embolism: analysis of the national registry. *Am J Obstet Gynecol* 1995;172:1158–67; discussion 1167-9.
7. Benson MD, Lindberg RE. Amniotic fluid embolism, anaphalxis, and tryptase. *Am J Obstet Gynecol* 1996;175:737.
8. Khong TY. Expression of endothelin-1 in amniotic fluid embolism and possible pathophysiological mechanism. *Br J Obstet Gynaecol* 1998;105:802–4.
9. Clark SL. New concepts of amniotic fluid embolism: a review. *Obstet Gynecol Surv* 1990;45:360–8.
10. Clarke SL, Pavlova Z, Greenspoon J, Horenstein J, Phelan JP. Squamous cells in the maternal pulmonary circulation. *Am J Obstet Gynecol* 1986;154:104–6.
11. Clarke SL, Cotton DB, Gonik B, Greenspoon J, Phelan JP. Central hemodynamic alterations in amniotic fluid embolism. *Am J Obstet Gynecol* 1988;158:1124–6.
12. Girard P, Mal H, Laine JF, Petitpretz P, Rain B, Duroux P. Left heart failure in amniotic fluid embolism. *Anesthesiology* 1986;64:262–5.
13. Lockwood CJ, Bach R, Guha A, Zhou XD, Miller WA, Nemerson Y. Amniotic fluid contains tissue factor, a potent initiator of coagulation. *Am J Obstet Gynecol* 1991;165:1335–41.
14. Stafford I, Sheffield J. Amniotic fluid embolism. *Obstet Gynecol Clin North Am* 2007;34:545–53, xii.

15. Dorairajan G, Soundararaghaven S. Maternal death after intrapartum saline amnioinfusion – report of two cases. *BJOG* 2005;112:1331–3.
16. Kramer MS, Rouleau J, Baskett TF, Joseph KS; Maternal Health Study Group of the Canadian Perinatal Surveillance System. Amniotic fluid embolism and medical induction of labour: a retrospective, population-based cohort study. *Lancet* 2006;368:1444–8.
17. Weiwen Y, Niugyu Z, Lauxiang Z, Yu L. Study of the diagnosis and management of amniotic fluid embolism: 38 cases of analysis. *Obstet Gynecol* 2000;95 Suppl:38S.
18. Margarson MP. Delayed amniotic fluid embolism following caesarean section under spinal anaesthesia. *Anaesthesia* 1995;50:804–6.
19. Kobayashi H, Ooi H, Hayakawa H, Arai T, Matsuda Y, Gotoh K, et al. Histological diagnosis of amniotic fluid embolism by monoclonal antibody TKH-2 that recognizes NeuAc alpha 2-6GalNac epitope. *Hum Pathol* 1997;28:428–33.
20. Benson MD, Kobayashi H, Silver RK, Oi H, Greenberger PA, Terao T. Immunologic studies in presumed amniotic fluid embolism. *Obstet Gynecol* 2001;97:510–4.
21. Kanckoy Y, Ogihara T, Tajima H, Mochimaru F. Continuous hemodiafiltration for disseminated intravascular coagulation and shock due to amniotic fluid embolism: report of a dramatic response. *Intern Med* 2001;40:945–7.
22. Tuffnell DJ. United Kingdom amniotic fluid embolism register. *BJOG* 2005;112:1625–9.

22 Disseminated intravascular coagulation

Disseminated intravascular coagulation (DIC), also known as consumptive coagulopathy, is a syndrome characterised by abnormal coagulation and fibrinolysis. DIC is acquired secondary to certain complications of pregnancy. A more detailed definition has been proposed by Bick: 'A systemic thrombohemorrhagic disorder seen in association with well-defined clinical situations and laboratory evidence of (a) procoagulant activation, (b) fibrinolytic activation, (c) inhibitor consumption, and (d) biochemical evidence of end-organ damage or failure.'[1]

Pathophysiology

Haemostasis is a dynamic balance between coagulation, which leads to fibrin formation, and fibrinolysis, which disposes of the fibrin once it has performed its coagulation function. During normal pregnancy there are progressive and profound changes in both of these systems.[2] The pro-coagulation factors 5, 7, 8, 9, 10, 12 and von Willebrand's factor all rise significantly. Fibrinogin levels are increased two-fold. These pro-coagulation changes, along with the increased blood volume, prepare the woman for blood loss at delivery and serve to produce haemostasis at the large uterine site of the separated placenta.

In DIC, there is excessive and generalised coagulation owing to the release of tissue thromboplastins into the maternal circulation. This causes excessive consumption and eventually depletion of the coagulation factors. Secondary to this widespread coagulation and deposition of fibrin in the microvasculature, the fibrinolytic system is activated. The breakdown of fibrin forms fibrin degradation products (FDP) which inhibit both fibrin and platelet function, aggravating the coagulation defect. The bleeding diathesis produced by this consumptive coagulopathy is the main element of DIC. In a smaller number of cases there is also widespread microvascular thrombosis leading to organ ischaemia and infarction, which, allied to the haemorrhagic shock, lead to the clinical manifestations of lung damage, renal cortical necrosis and/or Sheehan's syndrome.[3]

Causes

In pregnant women, DIC is always secondary to another obstetric complication. There are three main categories of conditions that may initiate DIC in pregnancy:[4]

- release of tissue factor into the maternal circulation
- injury to vascular endothelium
- red blood cell and/or platelet injury.

RELEASE OF TISSUE FACTOR (THROMBOPLASTINS) INTO THE MATERNAL CIRCULATION

The most common source of tissue factor in the maternal circulation is disrupted placental and decidual tissue from conditions such as placental abruption, amniotic fluid embolism, placenta accreta and uterine rupture. In such cases, the development of DIC is an acute manifestation. More rarely, insidious changes of DIC can develop in up to 25% of women with a retained dead fetus or delayed miscarriage of greater than 6 weeks' duration. In modern obstetrics, with early diagnosis by ultrasound, these more chronic causes of DIC are rare.

INJURY TO VASCULAR ENDOTHELIUM

Injury to vascular endothelium may expose the underlying collagen to plasma and coagulation factors. This can be the initiating cause of DIC in some women with eclampsia/pre-eclampsia, sepsis and hypovolaemic shock.

RED BLOOD CELL AND/OR PLATELET INJURY

Red blood cell and/or platelet injury can occur in response to massive blood transfusion, incompatible blood transfusion and septicaemia, leading to the release of procoagulant phospholipids.

In a number of obstetric complications, such as placental abruption, there may be interaction with one or all of the above mechanisms.

Clinical features

The main clinical features are usually those of the obstetric complication that precipitates the DIC. The haemorrhagic manifestations range from the subtle, including bruising, purpuric rash and venipuncture site oozing, to an obviously severe haemorrhagic diathesis with bleeding from all surgical sites and relentless postpartum haemorrhage.

The microvascular thrombotic sequelae are initially overshadowed by the above haemorrhagic features. If the woman survives, the most common thrombotic manifestations are hepatic, pulmonary and renal dysfunction.

Diagnosis

The diagnosis of DIC is usually based on the above clinical features allied to a variety of haematological tests. It is emphasised, however, that the process of DIC is so dynamic that the interpretation of test results can be difficult as they constantly change and, when received, may not reflect the current haematological state of the woman. When possible, consultation with a haematologist is desirable in these cases. The following tests may be of assistance:

- Both the prothrombin time and thrombin time are usually prolonged, although they can be normal.

- The partial thromboplastin time may be normal early in the process and only become prolonged late when the coagulation factors are severely depleted.

- Progressively falling platelet levels.

- The serum fibrinogen level is usually increased in pregnancy to 400–650 mg/dl. The level falls with DIC but may remain in the normal non-pregnant range. In severe DIC, the serum fibrinogen usually falls below 150 mg/dl. FDP are produced with DIC. Levels above 80 micrograms/dl confirm the diagnosis. Both FDP and D-dimer are elevated in the majority of cases. Even after the process of DIC has been controlled, elevated levels may remain for 24–48 hours.

- As red blood cells are forced through the fibrin mesh in the micro-vasculature, they become abnormally shaped and fragmented. A blood smear may show these abnormally shaped 'schistocytes'.

- If there is widespread destruction of red cells, microangiopathic haemolytic anaemia will ensue, resulting in haemolysis and haemo-globinuria.

Management

In a number of cases it may be possible to pre-empt the development of severe DIC with early intervention and management of the obstetric cause. Examples of this include the evacuation of the uterus in cases of fetal death and delayed miscarriage. It may also be possible in women with severe pre-eclampsia/HELLP syndrome (haemolysis, elevated liver enzymes, low platelets) and early changes of DIC. In such cases, prompt stabilisation of the mother and delivery of the fetus should prevent further deterioration into severe DIC.

However, in most obstetric situations DIC develops rapidly, so prompt and decisive treatment is required. There are three main principles of management: treat the initiating cause, maintain circulation and organ perfusion and replace procoagulants.

TREAT THE INITIATING CAUSE

DIC is always secondary to an obstetric cause and this should be sought and treated. These are covered in other chapters in this book, but in most cases the treatment entails emptying the uterus and/or controlling haemorrhage.

MAINTAIN CIRCULATION AND ORGAN PERFUSION

It is important to maintain an effective circulation to avoid tissue ischaemia and hypoxia. In addition, this process helps to clear the FDP which interfere with platelet function and have an antithrombin effect, thus compounding the DIC.

- Oxygen by face mask: endotracheal intubation and ventilation may be required.
- Rapid infusion of intravenous crystalloid, colloid and packed red blood cells.
- If facilities are available, monitor the circulation with a central venous pressure line. If not, try and keep the haematocrit greater than 30% and the urinary output more than 30 ml/hour.

REPLACE PROCOAGULANTS

The following principles can be used for the restoration of procoagulants:[5]

- Fresh frozen plasma contains all of the clotting factors, except platelets. The guiding principle is to give one unit of fresh frozen plasma after the initial transfusion of five units of blood. Thereafter, one unit of fresh frozen plasma is given for every two units of packed red blood cells transfused.
- Cryoprecipitate is rich in fibrinogen, von Willebrand's factor and factors 8 and 13. It is given for severe hypofibrinogenaemia.
- Severe thrombocytopenia (under 30 000/microlitre) may require platelet transfusion. Each unit of platelets will raise the count by approximately 5000–10 000/microlitre.

- Antithrombin is rapidly depleted by severe DIC. If levels are low, antithrombin concentrate may be given under the guidance of a haematologist.

- If coagulation is not restored by the above measures, recombinant activated factor VIIa should be considered. This factor combines with tissue factor to promote thrombin generation and stabilise fibrin formation. The dose is 60–80 mg/kg given intravenously. Recombinant activated factor VIIa is expensive and has a short half-life, but increasing experience in obstetric DIC confirms its value in selected cases.[5–8]

In obstetric DIC a guiding principle and a source of comfort is that the vast majority of these testing cases are in young healthy women who, provided the initiating cause is removed and their circulation and organ perfusion is maintained through the crisis, will recover completely.

References

1. Bick RL. Disseminated intravascular coagulation: a review of etiology, pathophysiology, diagnosis, and management: guidelines for care. *Clin Appl Thromb Hemost* 2002;8:1–31.
2. Brenner B. Haemostatic changes in pregnancy. *Thromb Res* 2004;114:409–14.
3. Levi M. Current understanding of disseminated intravascular coagulation. *Br J Haematol* 2004;124:567–76.
4. Williams J, Mosurkewich E, Chilimigras J, Van De Ven C. Critical care in obstetrics: pregnancy-specific conditions. *Best Pract Res Clin Obstet Gynaecol* 2008;22:825–46.
5. Searle E, Pavord S, Alfirevic Z. Recombinant factor VIIa and other pro-haemostatic therapies in primary postpartum haemorrhage. *Best Pract Res Clin Obstet Gynaecol* 2008;22:1075–88.
6. Alfirevic Z, Elbourne D, Pavord S, Bolte A, Van Geijn H, Mercier F, et al. Use of recombinant activated factor VII in primary postpartum haemorrhage: the Northern European registry 2000–2004. *Obstet Gynecol* 2007;110:1270–8.
7. Franchini M, Franchi M, Bergamini V, Montagnana M, Salvagno GL, Targher G, et al. The use of recombinant activated FVII in postpartum hemorrhage. *Clin Obstet Gynecol* 2010;53:219–27.
8. Karalapillai D, Popham P. Recombinant factor VIIa in massive postpartum haemorrhage. *Int J Obstet Anesth* 2007;16:29–34.

23 Acute tocolysis

As noted in other chapters, there are a number of conditions in obstetrics in which prompt relaxation of the uterus is necessary. In the past this could be achieved only by the rapid induction of general anaesthesia using halogenated agents, with its attendant risks. The development of simply administered tocolytic drugs has reduced the need for this risky use of general anaesthesia.

When acute tocolysis is required, regional anaesthesia in the form of spinal or epidural block may be in place. Although these regional anaesthetics provide good analgesia, they have no tocolytic effect; hence, the administration of tocolytic drugs is necessary to achieve optimum uterine relaxation.

Indications

EXCESSIVE UTERINE ACTION IN LABOUR

Uterine hyperstimulation in labour is defined as more than five uterine contractions in a 10-minute period (tachysystole) or contractions exceeding 2 minutes in duration (hypertonus).[1] Although uterine hyperstimulation can occur in spontaneous labour, it is more likely in pathological conditions such as placental abruption. Uterine hyperstimulation is most often found in response to uterotonic drugs such as oxytocin and, more commonly, prostaglandins which are used for cervical ripening and induction of labour.[2–4]

BREECH DELIVERY

At the time of caesarean delivery for breech presentation, when the fetal trunk has been delivered through the uterine incision, the uterus may contract down around the after-coming fetal head – rather like a tightly fitted helmet. This is particularly likely in the case of the premature infant in whom the head is much larger than the trunk. This can cause asphyxia owing to delay, and trauma to the fetal head, unless uterine relaxation is rapidly achieved.[5,6] Short-term tocolysis may also be used to facilitate external cephalic version of breech presentation at term.[7]

TWIN DELIVERY

After delivery of the first twin, external cephalic version or internal podalic version and breech extraction may be necessary to deliver the second twin (see chapter 12, page 148). For this to be safely carried out, the uterus must be completely relaxed.

SHOULDER DYSTOCIA WITH CEPHALIC REPLACEMENT

In the very rare instance of severe shoulder dystocia that cannot be resolved by other means, cephalic replacement may be considered (see chapter 10, page 127). In such cases, replacement of the head into the uterus may be facilitated by acute uterine relaxation. In addition, relaxation of the uterine muscle may improve uteroplacental blood flow and fetal oxygenation while delivery by caesarean section is being organised.

CORD PROLAPSE

If uterine contractions interfere with the ability to provide cord decompression in cases of cord prolapse, tocolysis may be indicated. This is usually necessary only if delay in performing caesarean delivery is anticipated (see chapter 17, page 191).

RETAINED PLACENTA

Relaxation of a contraction ring that is causing retention of a separated placenta may allow delivery of the placenta by controlled cord traction. In cases where the placenta has not separated, relaxation of the contraction ring should allow access of the hand for manual removal.[8]

ACUTE UTERINE INVERSION

In cases of acute uterine inversion, tocolysis may facilitate manual replacement of the uterus.[9]

Tocolytics

GLYCERYL TRINITRATE

Glyceryl trinitrate is an ester of nitric acid which is rapidly metabolised by the liver and has a half-life of 2–2.5 minutes. It has a low molecular weight (227 g/mol) and crosses the placenta, but there have been no adverse fetal or neonatal effects associated with its use. Glyceryl trinitrate causes peripheral vasodilatation and reduced venous tone, so significant maternal hypotension may occur.

Glyceryl trinitrate can be given by the sublingual or intravenous routes. Sublingual administration is usually via an aerosol, with two puffs equivalent to 800 micrograms.[10] However, mucosal absorption is variable and therefore the more precise intravenous route is usually chosen. An ampoule of glyceryl trinitrate contains 5 mg in 1 ml solution. A practical method for administration is to add this ampoule to a 100 ml bag of normal saline, which yields a solution of 50 micrograms/ml. Drawing up 20 ml into a syringe thus allows the precise administration of 50 micrograms/ml given. The peripheral vasodilatation effect of glyceryl trinitrate can be reversed with epinephrine (adrenaline) and the tocolytic effect responds to oxytocin.[11]

BETA-ADRENERGIC AGENTS

Beta-adrenergic agents are selective beta-2 receptor agonists. Their main effect is to relax arterial and uterine smooth muscle. The tocolytic effect usually lasts for 15–30 minutes. As such, beta-adrenergic agents may also cause hypotension and tachycardia, and there have been isolated reports of atrial fibrillation. These agents cross the placenta and can cause mild fetal tachycardia.

The two main drugs used for acute tocolysis in this category are terbutaline and hexoprenaline.[12,13]

ATOSIBAN

Atosiban is a synthetic analogue of oxytocin which binds to myometrial cell oxytocin receptors, acting as an oxytocin antagonist. Atisoban has a short half-life (12 minutes) and crosses the placenta without reported fetal or neonatal adverse effects. It has been used mainly to suppress preterm labour but may also have application for acute tocolysis in cases of uterine hypertonus causing fetal distress.[14–17]

Administration of tocolytic drugs

For cases of uterine hyperstimulation or abnormalities of the fetal heart rate in response to normal uterine labour contractions, the beta-adrenergic drugs or atosiban may be chosen.[15]

- Terbutaline can be given as 250 micrograms subcutaneously or at the same dose in 5 ml saline given intravenously over 5 minutes. The antagonist to terbutaline is propanolol 1–2 mg intravenously.

- Hexoprenaline is administered as 5 micrograms in 10 ml saline intravenously given over 5 minutes.

- Atosiban can be given intravenously over 1 minute as 6.75 mg in 5 ml normal saline.

- Glyceryl trinitrate is the drug of choice for acute tocolysis of brief duration necessary for the manipulations associated with breech and twin delivery, cephalic replacement and manual removal of the placenta. It is important to have intravenous crystalloid running rapidly to help fill the dilated intravascular space and avoid maternal hypotension.[18,19] The dose is titrated to match the clinical situation and the initial response.

In cases of fetal entrapment or cephalic replacement, rapid action is needed. One can start with an initial dose of glyceryl trinitrate 200 micrograms and repeat this at 1–2-minute intervals until adequate uterine relaxation occurs.

In women with retained placenta or acute uterine inversion, it is important to correct any associated hypovolaemia first. In this situation, a more graduated use of glyceryl trinitrate should be undertaken, usually starting with an initial dose of 100 micrograms and increasing according to the response. If the woman has previously received oxytocin or prostaglandins, higher doses of glyceryl trinitrate may be required.

In all the above clinical situations, the amount of drug given is a very individual titration of dose up to that required for appropriate uterine relaxation and should be balanced against maternal hypotension.

References

1. National Collaborating Centre for Women's and Children's Health, National Institute for Health and Clinical Excellence. *Induction of labour. Clinical Guideline.* London: RCOG Press; 2008.
2. Ingemarsson I, Arulkumaran S, Ratnam SS. Single injection of terbutaline in term labor. I. Effect on fetal pH in cases with prolonged bradycardia. *Am J Obstet Gynecol* 1985;153:859–65.
3. Ingemarsson I, Arulkumaran S, Ratnam SS. Single injection of terbutaline in term labor. II. Effect on uterine activity. *Am J Obstet Gynecol* 1985;153:865–9.
4. Palomäki O, Jansson M, Huhtala H, Kirkinen P. Severe cardiotocographic pathology at labor: effect of acute intravenous tocolysis. *Am J Perinatol* 2004;21:347–53.
5. Ezra Y, Wade C, Rolbin SH, Farine D. Uterine tocolysis at cesarean breech delivery with epidural anesthesia. *J Reprod Med* 2002;47:555–8.
6. Craig S, Dalton R, Tuck M, Brew F. Sublingual glyceryl trinitrate for uterine

relaxation at caesarean section – a prospective trial. *Aust N Z J Obstet Gynaecol* 1998;38:34–9.

7. Burgos J, Eguiguren N, Quintana E, Cobos P, Centeno M, Larrieta R, et al. Atosiban vs. ritodrine as a tocolytic in external cephalic version at term: a prospective cohort study. *J Perinat Med* 2010;38:23–8.

8. DeSimone CA, Norris MC, Leighton BL. Intravenous nitroglycerin aids manual extraction of a retained placenta. *Anesthesiology* 1990;73:787.

9. Altabef KM, Spencer JT, Zinberg S. Intravenous nitroglycerin for uterine relaxation of an inverted uterus. *Am J Obstet Gynecol* 1992;166:1237–8.

10. Clift K, Clift J. Uterine relaxation during caesarean section under regional anaesthesia: a survey of UK obstetric anaesthesists. *Int J Obstet Anesth* 2008;17:374–5.

11. Lau LC, Adaikan PG, Arulkumaran S, Ng SC. Oxytocics reverse the tocolytic effect of glyceryl trinitrate on the human uterus. *BJOG* 2001;108:164–8.

12. Shekarloo A, Mendez-Bauer C, Cook V, Freese U. Terbutaline (intravenous bolus) for the treatment of acute intrapartum fetal distress. *Am J Obstet Gynecol* 1989;160:615–8.

13. Chandraharan E, Arulkumaran S. Acute tocolysis. *Curr Opin Obstet Gynecol* 2005;17:151–6.

14. Afschar P, Schöll W, Bader A, Bauer M, Winter R. A prospective randomised trial of atosiban versus hexoprenaline for acute tocolysis and intrauterine resuscitation. *BJOG* 2004;111:316–8.

15. Chandraharan E, Arulkumaran S. Prevention of birth asphyxia: responding appropriately to cardiotocograph (CTG) traces. *Best Pract Res Clin Obstet Gynaecol* 2007;21:609–24.

16. de Heus R, Mulder EJ, Derks JB, Kurver PH, van Wolfswinkel L, Visser GH. A prospective randomized trial of acute tocolysis in term labour with atosiban or ritodrine. *Eur J Obstet Gynecol Reprod Biol* 2008;139:139–45.

17. de Heus R, Mulder EJ, Derks JB, Visser GH. Acute tocolysis for uterine activity reduction in term labor: a review. *Obstet Gynecol Surv* 2008;63:383–8.

18. Axemo P, Fu X, Lindberg B, Ulmstan U, Wessén A. Intravenous nitroglycerine for rapid uterine relaxation. *Acta Obstet Gynecol Scand* 1998;77:50–3.

19. O'Grady JP, Parker RK, Patel SS. Nitroglycerin for rapid tocolysis: development of a protocol and a literature review. *J Perinatol* 2000;20:27–33.

24 Severe pre-eclampsia and eclampsia

Hypertensive disease in pregnancy is a prominent cause of maternal and perinatal mortality and morbidity in both developed and developing countries. In regions with well-organised health services, the incidence of eclampsia is about 1/2000 maternities, with 1/200 women developing severe pre-eclampsia.[1] Although maternal death is rare in these countries, there is significant maternal and perinatal morbidity.[2,3] In developing countries, the incidence and mortality rates of eclampsia are about 20-fold higher, with maternal mortality rates of 15–20% and perinatal loss rates of about 20–40%.[4,5]

The definition of severe pre-eclampsia varies but is usually taken to be sustained hypertension greater than 160/100 mmHg associated with proteinuria over 1 g/litre. The addition of one or more convulsions defines eclampsia.

Conservative management of carefully selected cases of severe pre-eclampsia between 25 and 32 weeks of gestation may be considered to gain more time for fetal maturity.[6] This chapter covers management during labour or when the decision has been taken to terminate the pregnancy by induction of labour or caesarean section.

Clinical and pathological features

There are certain women who are at increased risk of developing pre-eclampsia.

PREDISPOSING FACTORS TO PRE-ECLAMPSIA

- Family history
- Primigravida
- Age less than 20 years and over 35 years
- Chronic hypertension or renal disease
- Diabetes mellitus
- Multiple pregnancy
- Gestational trophoblastic disease
- Antiphospholipid syndrome

Severe pre-eclampsia/eclampsia is a multi-organ disease process of undetermined aetiology. The clinical manifestations depend on the predominant end-organ involvement and effect.

CLINICAL FEATURES OF SEVERE PRE-ECLAMPSIA

- Sustained hypertension over 160/100 mmHg
- Proteinuria over 1 g/litre (2+ dipstick)
- ± Oedema

ADDITIONAL FEATURES

- Neurological
  - double or blurred vision
  - scotoma
  - frontal headache
  - hyperreflexia and sustained clonus
  - Oliguria
- Epigastric and right hypochondrial pain
- Nausea and vomiting
- Thrombocytopenia
- Abnormal liver function tests
- Pulmonary oedema
- Papilloedema

HYPERTENSION AND PROTEINURIA

The common underlying pathology in pre-eclampsia is vascular spasm resulting in hypertension. In severe pre-eclampsia, blood pressure exceeds 160/100 mmHg, although the degree of rise of blood pressure is also important. The young primigravid woman whose normal blood pressure is 90/60 mmHg may develop eclampsia with a blood pressure of less than 160/100 mmHg.

It is important to realise that automated methods of blood pressure recording can underestimate the degree of hypertension. Similarly, in an era of increasingly obese arms, a larger blood pressure cuff is often required. Korotkoff phase 5 is the appropriate measurement of diastolic blood pressure.[1] Multiple readings are taken with the woman sitting at a 45° angle.

Renal involvement is manifest by glomerular endotheliosis, in which the capillary endothelial cells are swollen, leading to glomerular ischaemia and reduced glomerular filtration. This leads to oliguria and proteinuria. In severe pre-eclampsia, the degree of proteinuria is at least

1 g/litre and often greater than 5 g in 24 hours. Although dipstick testing can be variable, clinical urgency often dictates that this is the only appraisal of the degree of proteinuria available, rather than the more accurate 24-hour urine collection. In such cases, dipstick 2+ equals 1 g/litre of proteinuria

The classical triad of pre-eclampsia is hypertension, proteinuria and oedema. However, in many cases oedema is absent or minimal. When present, oedema is usually most obvious in the face and hands. Occult fluid retention may be manifest by marked weight gain in the days or weeks before the development of severe pre-eclampsia.

CONVULSIONS

Convulsions represent the most dramatic manifestation and move the diagnosis from severe pre-eclampsia to eclampsia, worsening the prognosis for both mother and fetus. About 40% of cases of eclampsia are antepartum, 20% intrapartum and 40% postpartum. The seizure is of the grand mal type and thought to be caused by vasospasm of the cerebral arteries leading to ischaemia and cerebral oedema. Convulsions may be followed by coma, cortical blindness and focal motor deficits. In most cases these are transient.[7] Cerebrovascular haemorrhage complicates 1–2% of cases.[8]

Prodromal symptoms of eclampsia in the woman with severe pre-eclampsia include double or blurred vision, scotoma and frontal headache. Many women are also hyperreflexic, but this is too common a finding in women with pre-eclampsia to be a sensitive predictor of eclampsia.

HEPATIC INVOLVMENT

Vasospasm in the vascular bed of the liver may be associated with intravascular fibrin deposition and periportal haemorrhagic necrosis. Liver enzymes are elevated and, on rare occasions, bleeding can occur beneath the liver capsule and rupture into the peritoneal cavity with catastrophic results.

PULMONARY OEDEMA

Pulmonary oedema occurs in fewer than 5% of cases of severe pre-eclampsia and is a result of a combination of factors including low colloid osmotic pressure, pulmonary capillary leak, left ventricular dysfunction and iatrogenic fluid overload.

HAEMATOLOGICAL MANIFESTATIONS

The hypercoagulable state of all pregnant women is accentuated in pre-eclampsia. This may be a result of vasospasm in the vasa vasorum leading to hypoxia and damage of the endothelial walls in the micro-vasculature. Thus, a low level of disseminated intravascular coagulation (DIC) may occur, with the most common manifestation being thrombocytopenia (see chapter 22, page 242). Mild thrombocytopenia (under 100 000 ml) is not uncommon, but the full picture of microangiopathic haemolytic anaemia or DIC is rare.

HELLP SYNDROME

Within the clinical spectrum of severe pre-eclampsia/eclampsia is the HELLP syndrome (haemolysis, elevated liver enzymes and low platelets). HELLP syndrome was first described in 1982 and complicates 4–12% of cases of severe pre-eclampsia/eclampsia.[9] HELLP syndrome may present a very wide clinicopathological spectrum, ranging from a gastrointestinal presentation with nausea, vomiting and right upper quadrant pain, mimicking gall bladder disease and without hypertension, to a florid case with severe pre-eclampsia/eclampsia, jaundice, DIC and severe thrombocytopenia.[10]

FETAL EFFECTS

Uteroplacental blood flow, and therefore perfusion of the intervillus space, is often reduced in women with severe pre-eclampsia/eclampsia. This may present as fetal growth restriction and/or hypoxia. Placental abruption is also more common in these women.

Management

MANAGEMENT OF SEVERE PRE-ECLAMPSIA/ECLAMPSIA
● Protect and maintain airway
● Stop or prevent convulsions
● Treat hypertension/cardiovascular monitoring
● Fluid balance/monitor renal function
● Detection and management of thrombocytopenia and disseminated intravascular coagulation
● Deliver the fetus: induction of labour/caesarean section

ANTICONVULSANT THERAPY

Since the Collaborative Eclampsia Trial[11] in the 1990s, magnesium sulphate has been established as the treatment of choice for prevention of convulsions in women with eclampsia. Magnesium sulphate prophylaxis should also be given to women with severe pre-eclampsia as it has been shown to be superior to placebo in randomised trials.[12,13]

Magnesium sulphate acts as a vasodilator and as a membrane stabiliser; it may also have a central anticonvulsant effect. The initial dose of magnesium sulphate is 4 g by intravenous infusion over 20 minutes. A 50% solution of magnesium sulphate contains 1 g/2 ml. Thus, the loading dose is 8 ml of the 50% solution followed by a maintenance dose of 1–2 g/hour using a controlled infusion device. High levels of magnesium sulphate can cause fatal respiratory and cardiovascular depression. Careful monitoring of continued magnesium sulphate therapy is therefore required.

Biochemical monitoring is necessary only in cases of renal dysfunction with persistent oliguria. In such cases the aim is to keep the magnesium level between 2 mmol/l and 4 mmol/l (between 4 mg/dl and 8 mg/dl). In most instances biological monitoring is adequate. If the respiratory rate is less than 12/minute, deep tendon reflexes are absent (patella reflex if no epidural, biceps tendon if epidural in place) and oliguria is less than 25 ml/hour, the magnesium sulphate infusion should be stopped. The magnesium sulphate can be restarted at 1 g/hour when the respiratory rate has come back to normal and the deep tendon reflexes have returned. The presence of oliguria is very important as magnesium sulphate is excreted solely by the kidneys. In many cases a pulse oximeter is a useful aid.

If magnesium sulphate overdose occurs, as shown by the above biological features plus periods of apnoea and deep sedation, the antidote to magnesium sulphate, calcium gluconate 1 g (10 ml of 10% solution), should be given intravenously over 5 minutes. Occasionally, it may be necessary to support ventilation by mechanical means until the plasma magnesium sulphate levels have fallen.

If the woman is first seen during an eclamptic fit, the fit should be controlled by the bolus dose of magnesium sulphate previously described or with diazepam 10 mg intravenously over 1 minute. This should then be followed by magnesium sulphate prophylaxis, as outlined above.

If a woman on magnesium sulphate prophylaxis has a seizure, the seizure should be controlled with a 2 g bolus of magnesium sulphate given over 2–3 minutes or, if this fails, by diazepam 10 mg intravenously.

On rare occasions, the above anticonvulsant therapy is unsuccessful and these women may require a thiopentone drip, muscle relaxants, intubation and assisted ventilation in an intensive care unit.

ANTIHYPERTENSIVE THERAPY

The most serious risk to the mother from the hypertension of pre-eclampsia is cerebral haemorrhage. For this reason, hypotensive therapy should be given if the diastolic blood pressure is sustained at ≥110 mmHg. A balance has to be achieved between this goal and excessive reduction of the blood pressure, which may reduce uteroplacental blood flow and threaten the fetus. One therefore aims to reduce the blood pressure by 15–20% so that the systolic blood pressure is kept between 140 mmHg and 160 mmHg and the diastolic blood pressure is in the 90–100 mmHg range.

The following regimens are available:[14,15]

- Hydralazine, a peripheral vasodilator, is given as an initial dose of 5 mg intravenously over 2 minutes. Thereafter, doses of 5–10 mg can be given by intravenous bolus every 20 minutes as needed. Alternatively, a continuous intravenous infusion can be established at a dose of 5 mg/hour and adjusted accordingly. Tachycardia and headache, the results of vasodilatation, are common adverse effects, and tachyphylaxis can also occur.

- Labetalol, a combined alpha- and beta-adrenergic blocker, is administered intravenously at a dose of 20 mg, followed by 40 mg if ineffective in 15 minutes. A continuous infusion is then established and adjusted as necessary. The maximum total parenteral dose is 300 mg. The personnel looking after the baby should be aware that labetalol can cause neonatal bradycardia.

- Nifedipine is a calcium channel blocker which can be given by mouth. The dose is one 10 mg capsule orally every 30 minutes as required, up to a maximum of 80 mg. The capsule form should not be confused with the intermediate-release tablets and slow-release tablets of nifedipine.

All of the above regimens are acceptable, but it is a good idea for each unit to get accustomed to one routine and learn how to fine-tune the dosing to accommodate individual cases. In many hospitals labetalol is chosen, especially if the mother has tachycardia.

FLUID BALANCE/CARDIOVASCULAR MONITORING

Plasma volume is decreased in severe pre-eclampsia. However, the available intravascular space is filled and these women do not tolerate haemorrhage or the loss of fluid from diuretic administration. On the other hand, attempts to expand the blood volume with intravenous fluid may overload the circulation. Along with the reduced colloid osmotic pressure associated with hypoalbuminaemia, these women are very vulnerable to pulmonary oedema. If the vasoconstriction is relaxed by hypotensive agents or epidural regional anaesthesia, additional intravenous fluid will be required to fill the expanded intravascular space. The aim, therefore, is to provide intravenous crystalloid to cover the insensible loss and urinary output, and also to provide more intravenous fluid if the intravascular space is expanded by hypotensive drugs or regional anaesthesia.

While it is not necessary in all cases, a central venous pressure line may be of assistance in guiding this fluid management.[16] The aim is to keep the central venous pressure value between 4 mmHg and 8 mmHg. An initial intravenous infusion of 100 ml/hour is reasonable. One must remember that the fluids infusing the anticonvulsants and hypotensive medications must be included in this figure. An indwelling Foley catheter is required to monitor the urinary output, which should ideally be greater than 25 ml/hour. It may be necessary to monitor left ventricular function with a Swan–Ganz catheter if the hypertension is severe and hard to control, if there is marked oliguria or if pulmonary oedema develops. In these cases the guidance of those regularly involved with intensive care is required and the assistance of the obstetric anaesthetist is essential.

HAEMATOLOGICAL CONSIDERATIONS

The most common abnormality is thrombocytopenia, which is present if the platelet count is less than 100 000/ml. Spontaneous haemorrhage is unlikely to occur unless the level falls below 20 000/ml. However, if caesarean section is required, platelet transfusion may be necessary to keep the count greater than 50 000/ml. If thrombocytopenia develops, the other criteria of the HELLP syndrome should be sought. The rare development of DIC requires the management outlined in chapter 22 (page 241).

ANALGESIA AND ANAESTHESIA

If available, epidural analgesia is desirable for pain relief in labour and for operative vaginal or caesarean delivery. The absence of pain, and its associated catecholamine rise, helps control the blood pressure. Greater control of maternal bearing-down effort is also desirable to minimise hypertension. For the reasons mentioned above, epidural anaesthesia will increase the intravascular space and may be associated with acute hypotension unless appropriate preloading with intravenous crystalloid is carried out.

General anaesthesia may be required if there is a coagulopathy, but this carries increased risks in the presence of laryngeal oedema, making intubation difficult or even impossible, as well as having the potential to worsen laryngeal oedema and cause postoperative respiratory obstruction. In addition, during induction and recovery from anaesthesia and intubation, there is a transient exacerbation of hypertension.

CLINICAL/NURSING CARE

Women with severe pre-eclampsia/eclampsia require intensive nursing care and the close supervision of an experienced obstetric consultant. An obstetric anaesthestist should be involved early on during induction and/or labour. Depending on the complexity of the case and the type of complications, the assistance of other consultants, such as internal medicine, haematology and renal medicine, may be necessary.

The woman should be nursed in a single quiet room with a mouth gag readily available at the bedside to place between the jaws and protect the tongue should an eclamptic convulsion occur.

During the initial loading dose of antihypertensive medication, the blood pressure should be recorded every 5 minutes. Thereafter, blood pressure can be taken every 15–30 minutes as the pressure stabilises. The woman's reflexes, respiratory rate, fluid balance and urinary output should be recorded hourly. If applicable, central venous pressure and oxygen saturation should also be recorded hourly.

DELIVERY

The only cure for severe pre-eclampsia/eclampsia is delivery of the fetus and placenta. The treatment outlined up to now is aimed at protecting the mother and fetus until delivery can be accomplished.

If conditions are favourable for induction of labour, this is the treatment of choice with amniotomy and oxytocin. If the cervix is unfavourable but maternal and fetal condition are stable and well controlled, the use of vaginal prostaglandins to induce labour may be acceptable. If time permits, and the gestation is less than 34 weeks, two 12 mg intramuscular doses of betamethasone may be given 12 hours apart.

Caesarean section is chosen if there are other obstetric indications such as breech presentation, fetal growth restriction, cases that are very unfavourable for induction or non-progressive labour.

As mentioned above, epidural anaesthesia is the ideal for labour and vaginal delivery. Appropriate use of oxytocin augmentation during the second stage of labour should allow the head to deliver spontaneously with minimal maternal effort or by assisted low pelvis delivery, either by forceps or by vacuum. Oxytocin should be used for management of the third stage of labour. Ergometrine is specifically contraindicated because of its tendency to precipitate a hypertensive crisis in these women.

POSTPARTUM

Anticonvulsant therapy should continue for at least 24 hours after delivery or after the last convulsion, whichever is the longer time period. During this time the woman should continue to be treated in an intensive obstetric area with continuous nursing care. Usually, the antihypertensive therapy can be reduced postpartum, but occasionally an oral hypotensive agent may be needed for the first 2–4 weeks postpartum. Thrombocytopenia, if present, tends to reach its nadir 24–30 hours postpartum and then spontaneously recover. A diuresis, which is often quite profound, usually occurs within 12–24 hours.

Severe pre-eclampsia is not common and eclampsia is rare in developed countries. Even large obstetric units may see only up to two eclamptic cases per year. It is necessary for all obstetric units to have guidelines and protocols for the management of these cases. Consistent application of these guidelines and early involvement of experienced medical and nursing staff is essential to ensure the best outcome.

Before the woman is discharged from hospital, the future outlook for her own health and for subsequent pregnancies should be discussed. The woman has approximately a 10–20% chance of developing pre-eclampsia in another pregnancy. This advice can be fine-tuned depending on the presence of other factors, such as chronic hypertension, antiphospholipid syndrome and so on.

References

1. Royal College of Obstetricians and Gynaecologists. *The management of severe pre-eclampsia/eclampsia*. Green-top Guideline No. 10(A). London: RCOG; 2006 [http://www.rcog.org.uk/womens-health/clinical-guidance/management-severe-pre-eclampsiaeclampsia-green-top-10a].
2. Lee W, O'Connell CM, Baskett TF. Maternal and perinatal outcomes of eclampsia: Nova Scotia, 1981–2000. *J Obstet Gynaecol Can* 2004;26:119–23.
3. Tuffnell DJ, Jankowicz D, Lindow SW, Lyons G, Mason GC, Russel IF, et al.; Yorkshire Obstetric Critical Care Group. Outcomes of severe pre-eclampsia/eclampsia in Yorkshire 1999/2003. *BJOG* 2005;112:875–80.
4. Olatunji AO, Sule Odu AO. Maternal mortality from eclampsia. *J Obstet Gynaecol* 2006;26:542–3.
5. Igberase GO, Ebeigbe PN. Eclampsia: ten-years of experience in a rural tertiary hospital in the Niger delta, Nigeria. *J Obstet Gynaecol* 2006;26:414–7.

6. Hall DR, Odendall HJ, Steyn DW, Grové D. Expectant management of early onset, severe pre-eclampsia: maternal outcome. *BJOG* 2000;107:1252–7.
7. Arulkumaran S, Gibb DM, Rauff M, Kek LP, Ratnam SS. Transient blindness associated with pregnancy-induced hypertension. Case reports. *Br J Obstet Gynaecol* 1985,92:847–9.
8. Douglas KA, Redman CW. Eclampsia in the United Kingdom. *BMJ* 1994;309:1395–400.
9. Weinstein L. Syndrome of hemolysis, elevated liver enzymes and low platelet count: a severe consequence of hypertension in pregnancy. *Am J Obstet Gynecol* 1982;142:159–67.
10. Sibai BM. Diagnosis, controversies, and management of the syndrome of hemolysis, elevated liver enzymes, and low platelet count. *Obstet Gynecol* 2004;103:981–91.
11. Which anticonvulsant for women with eclampsia? Evidence from the Collaborative Eclampsia Trial. *Lancet* 1995;345:1455–63.
12. Altman D, Carroli G, Duley L, Farrell B, Moodley J, Neilson J, et al.; Magpie Trial Collaboration Group. Do women with pre-eclampsia, and their babies, benefit from magnesium sulphate? The Magpie Trial: a randomised placebo-controlled trial. *Lancet* 2002;359:1877–90.
13. Sibai BM. Diagnosis, prevention, and management of eclampsia. *Obstet Gynecol* 2005;105:402–10.
14. Magee LA, Chan C, Waterman EJ, Ohlsson A, von Dadelszen P. Hydralazine for treatment of severe hypertension in pregnancy: meta-analysis. *BMJ* 2003;327:9550–60.
15. Magee LA, Helewa M, Moutquin JM, von Dadelszen P. Treatment of the hypertensive disorders of pregnancy. *J Obstet Gynaecol Can* 2008;30 Suppl 1:S24–36.
16. Young P, Johanson R. Haemodynamic, invasive and echocardiographic monitoring in the hypertensive parturient. *Clin Obstet Gynaecol* 2001;15:605–22.

25 Neonatal resuscitation

Only 1–2% of newborns will require active resuscitation. Anticipation of deliveries where problems may occur, rapid and systematic assessment of the newborn and application of practical resuscitation techniques are required by those attending deliveries.[1-3]

Examples of cases that may require resuscitation include:

- emergency caesarean deliveries
- breech presentation
- fetal distress/perinatal asphyxia
- meconium aspiration syndrome
- expected major fetal abnormality (such as congenital diaphragmatic hernia)
- preterm deliveries (at less than 35 completed weeks of gestation).

Before any assessment, it is important to dry and cover the baby to prevent heat loss.

Assessment

While the Apgar score has traditionally been used to evaluate babies in need of resuscitation (Table 25.1), a rapid assessment of heart rate and breathing is most useful in determining the need for active resuscitation. This should take no longer than 30 seconds.

Table 25.1 The Agpar scoring system			
Measure score	*0*	*1*	*2*
Heart rate	Absent	<100 bpm	>100 bpm
Respiratory effort	Absent	Slow, irregular	Regular with crying
Muscle tone	Limp	Some tone in limbs	Active flexion
Reflex irritability	Nil	Grimace only	Vigorous crying
Colour	Pale	Pink with blue extremities	Pink

Heart rate may be assessed by auscultation or by palpation of the base of the umbilical cord. A normal heart rate is above 100 beats/minute. If a pulse oximeter is readily available, this is the most reliable way of assessing heart rate and oxygen saturation following delivery, but resuscitation should not be delayed to set this up.

Breathing may be assessed visually, looking for chest movement. Most babies establish breathing by about 90 seconds of age.

Following assessment, babies can be broadly categorised into three main categories:

- healthy
- apnoeic
- freshly stillborn.

HEALTHY BABIES

Following drying, a healthy baby will have good tone, a heart rate above 100 beats/minute and regular breathing/crying.

ACTION: Wrap warmly and give to mother.

APNOEIC BABIES

Apnoea may be primary or secondary/terminal. Following a hypoxic event in utero, the fetus will attempt to breathe. If hypoxia continues, the fetus will become apnoeic owing to central suppression of respiration (primary apnoea). After a pause, primitive spinal reflexes trigger further gasping; however, with continued hypoxia these reflexes eventually cease and the fetus again becomes apnoeic (terminal apnoea) and will not re-initiate breathing without external intervention. The heart rate will be present, but will be less than 100 beats/minute.

It is not possible to reliably judge whether a baby is in primary or terminal apnoea during the initial assessment, although some babies in primary apnoea may respond to gentle stimulation.

ACTION: Gentle stimulation by drying/ rubbing the back. If there is no response within 30 seconds, proceed to A B C D as described below.

FRESHLY STILLBORN BABIES

Freshly stillborn babies are floppy and have no heart rate or breathing.

ACTION: Proceed to A B C D as described below.

The A B C D of resuscitation

- **A**irway: dry, warm, assess and position airway and stimulate to breathe.
- **B**reathing: inflation breaths and ventilation.
- **C**irculation: chest compressions.
- **D**rugs: medications and volume if required.

Each step should take approximately 30 seconds. Progression to the next step is dependent on successful completion of the previous step. There is an excellent algorithm published by the Resuscitation Council (UK)[3] (Figure 25.1).

Maintain temperature and assess: dry the baby, wrap in a warm towel and place on a flat surface. Use a resuscitaire if available, making sure the heater is on and the clock started. Then assess the baby (see above).

AIRWAY

The airway must be open before the baby can breathe effectively. Position the baby face upwards with the head in the neutral position (neither flexed nor extended, with face parallel with the resuscitation surface). Suction at this stage is not necessary unless there is obvious airway obstruction. If suctioning of the oropharynx is required, this should be performed under direct vision.

BREATHING

After positioning the airway, if the baby remains apnoeic, five inflation breaths should be given to inflate the lungs via a face mask (see below). Inflation breaths are longer than normal breaths and should last for 2–3 seconds at a pressure of 30 cm H_2O (20 cm H_2O in preterm infants). These breaths are required to aerate lungs that are filled with fluid. Current evidence suggests that air should be used in preference to oxygen during the initial resuscitation of term infants, as use of 100% oxygen delays the onset of spontaneous respiration and may be associated with increased mortality.[4–6]

Ventilation via a face mask

The mask should be large enough to cover the nose and mouth without pressing on the eyes (Figure 25.2). A self-inflating bag or T-piece ventilation system should be used for inflation breaths. Make sure that good contact is made so that an effective seal is created. Breaths are given

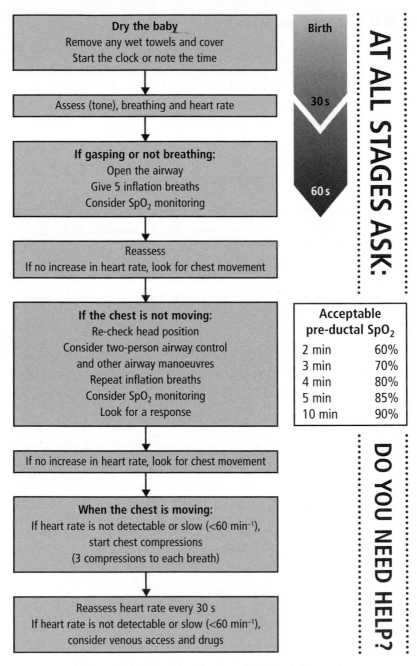

Figure 25.1 Algorithm for resuscitation of the newborn

Reproduced with permission from the Newborn Life Support guidelines (2010), Resuscitation Council (UK). s = seconds; SpO$_2$ = saturation of peripheral oxygen.

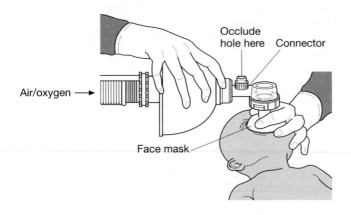

Figure 25.2 Neonatal resuscitation using a bag and mask

either by squeezing the self-inflating bag or by occluding the hole in the T-piece ventilation connector. Pressure is limited to 30–40 cm H_2O by a pressure blow-off valve in the self-inflating bag system, or by setting a pressure limit on the resuscitaire with the T-piece ventilation system. Some T-piece systems also allow the setting of a positive end-expiratory pressure (PEEP) to reduce alveolar collapse during ventilation. This is achieved either by adjusting the gas flow rate or by an adjustable screw fitting in the T-piece (Figure 25.3). It is important to be familiar with the

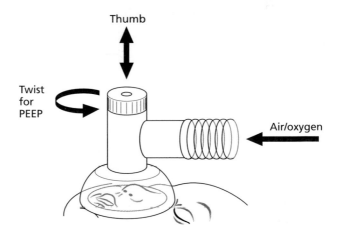

Figure 25.3 T-piece ventilation: occlude the hole with the thumb to give breath; in this model, twisting the end-piece controls the PEEP

PEEP = positive end-expiratory pressure.

system that you are using, as excessive PEEP may prevent adequate ventilation and may even cause harm.

A pressure of 30 cm H_2O is usually sufficient to provide adequate tidal volume in a term infant.

Inflation breaths can be judged to be successful when the heart rate increases to above 100 beats/minute or when chest rise is seen (the lower sternum will move 1–2 cm with each breath). Following successful inflation breaths, establish a rate of 30–40 breaths/minute. If the heart rate does not increase and the chest does not move, it is important to check the mask seal and return to airway before proceeding.

Trying a one- or two-person jaw thrust, or insertion of a Guedel airway, will establish airway patency in nearly all babies.

Intubation

Intubation requires considerable practice and is usually not required in the initial resuscitation period if adequate ventilation can be established via a mask.

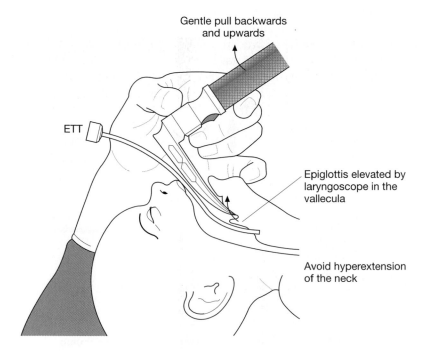

Figure 25.4 Using the laryngoscope to visualise the structures that allow correct placement of the endotracheal tube

Figure 25.4 illustrates use of the laryngoscope to visualise the structures that allow correct placement of the endotracheal tube. For small babies use a 2.5 mm endotracheal tube and for term babies a 3.0–3.5 mm endotracheal tube.

In term infants, aim for a rate of 30–40 breaths/minute at a pressure of 30 cm H_2O, with breaths lasting 0.5–1 second. The pressure can be increased to 40 cm H_2O if necessary.

To confirm that the endotracheal tube is in position following intubation, check for:

- a rise in/maintenance of heart rate and oxygen saturations
- carbon dioxide on expiration using a colorimetric carbon dioxide detector if available, in a baby with cardiac output: false negatives may occur in very small preterm babies, while false positives can occur if the device is contaminated with adrenaline, surfactant or atropine
- bilateral chest movement
- breath sounds that are equal bilaterally on auscultation
- absence of breath sounds over the stomach.

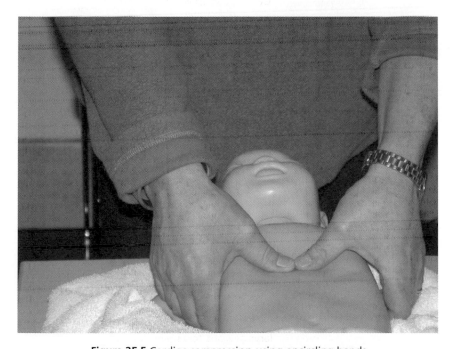

Figure 25.5 Cardiac compression using encircling hands

CIRCULATION

Cardiac compression

Once adequate ventilation has been established for 30 seconds, cardiac compressions should be commenced if the heart rate remains below 60 beats/minute. This may be performed in one of two ways:

• Encircle the chest so that the fingers lie behind the baby and the thumbs are opposed over the mid-sternum (Figure 25.5). This is the preferred method.

• Place two fingers over the sternum 1 cm below the inter-nipple line (Figure 25.6).

Compressions should be carried out at a ratio of three compressions to one ventilation breath at an event rate of 120/minute. Depress the sternum to a depth of 1–2 cm.

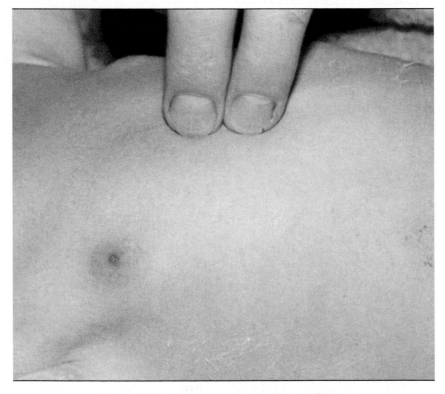

Figure 25.6 Cardiac compression using two fingers

Table 25.2 Drugs used in neonatal resuscitation

Drug	Dosage and route of administration	Comments
Adrenaline (epinephrine)	0.01–0.03 mg/kg (0.1–0.3 ml/kg of 1:10 000) IV. If IV access cannot be obtained, consider 0.05–0.1 mg/kg via ETT (0.5–1 ml/kg of 1: 10000).	The only drug routinely recommended in resuscitation.
Volume expansion	10–20 ml/kg IV over 10–20 seconds.	Early volume expansion in babies suspected of acute blood loss with 0.9% saline is recommended. This may be followed by rhesus-negative blood. If there is no response to ventilation and adrenaline, volume expansion may still be tried even in the absence of evidence of blood loss.
Sodium bicarbonate	0.5–1 mmol/kg (1–2 ml/kg of 4.2% solution) IV only. 8.4% bicarbonate should be diluted 1:1 with water for injection before administration.	Sodium bicarbonate can be tried if there is no response to adrenaline.
Naloxone		There is no role for naloxone in emergency neonatal resuscitation.

ETT = endotracheal tube; IV = intravenous

DRUGS

Drugs are rarely needed in neonatal resuscitation. They are indicated if adequate ventilation and effective cardiac compressions fail to increase the heart rate to above 60 beats/minute (Table 25.2).

Resuscitation of the baby with meconium-stained liquor

If a baby is vigorous following birth, evidence suggests that there is no role for suction of the oropharynx, whether meconium is present or not.[7] In the non-vigorous baby born through thick meconium, suctioning of the oropharynx and trachea under direct vision, and intubation before ventilation if personnel are skilled in this technique, can be tried. If intubation is unsuccessful or prolonged, especially in the presence of a falling or low heart rate, oxygen delivery becomes the most urgent priority and commencing mask ventilation may be life-saving.

Actions in the event of poor response to resuscitation

Following a structured approach of constant assessment using the A B C D approach will resuscitate the vast majority of newborn infants. Failure to respond may indicate a loss of airway patency, inadequate ventilation (such as a poor mask seal) or an incorrectly placed endotracheal tube.

Other causes to consider include:

- A technical fault:
  o Inadequate ventilation pressure being given: check the blow-off valve or T-piece pressure dial.
  o Inadvertently giving too high PEEP: check the T-piece pressure dial.
  o Endotracheal tube blocked or dislodged: if in any doubt, remove and either replace or revert to mask ventilation.
  o Baby requires an increased oxygen concentration.
- Lung pathology:
  o Pneumothorax.
  o Diaphragmatic hernia.
  o Hypoplastic lungs.
- If there is good chest movement, has there been:
  o Fetal haemorrhage? Consider volume expansion.
  o Severe asphyxia?

Resuscitation of the preterm infant

If available, preterm babies should be placed directly into a clear plastic bag without drying to prevent heat loss, but with the head exposed.[8] Preterm babies should be managed on a resuscitaire with the heater on if available. Lower pressures of 18–25 cm H_2O should be used initially, but the pressure may need to be increased if response is inadequate (heart rate fails to increase above 100 beats/minute or starts to fall, and chest movement is not seen). Early administration of surfactant may be indicated if intubation is required. The ideal oxygen concentration to use is unclear; however, a personal recommendation is to start at 30–40% and adjust according to response (heart rate and oxygen saturation).

Therapeutic hypothermia

There is clear evidence to support the use of therapeutic hypothermia in term infants with evidence of hypoxic ischaemic brain injury.[9] Hypothermia must be started in the first 6 hours of life if it is to be most effective, so early discussion with an appropriate specialist centre is advised.

When should resuscitation be stopped?

Babies who have no heart rate for more than 10 minutes are very unlikely to survive and, if they do survive, are very likely to have severe neurological disability. At this stage it is appropriate to consider stopping resuscitation. This should be a team decision, led by the most senior paediatrician present.[1–3]

References

1. Richmond S, Wyllie J. European Resuscitation Council Guidelines for Resuscitation 2010 Section 7. Resuscitation of babies at birth. *Resuscitation* 2010;81:1389–99.
2. Perlman JM, Wyllie J, Kattwinkel J, Atkins DL, Chameides L, Goldsmith JP, et al.; Neonatal Resuscitation Chapter Collaborators. Part 11: Neonatal resuscitation: 2010 International Consensus on Cardiopulmonary Resuscitation and Emergency Cardiovascular Care Science With Treatment Recommendations. *Circulation.* 2010;122 Suppl 2:S516–38.
3. Richmond S, Wyllie J. Newborn Life Support. In: Nolan JP, editor. *The Resuscitation Guidelines 2010.* London: Resuscitation Council (UK); 2010 [http://www.resus.org.uk/pages/guide.htm].
4. Davis PG, Tan A, O'Donnell CPF, Schulze A. Resuscitation of newborn infants with 100% oxygen or air: a systematic review and meta-analysis. *Lancet* 2004;364:1329–33.
5. Rabi Y, Rabi D, Yee W. Room air resuscitation of the depressed newborn: a systematic review and meta-analysis. *Resuscitation* 2007;72:353–63.
6. Saugstad OD, Ramji S, Vento M. Resuscitation of depressed newborn infants with ambient air or pure oxygen: a meta-analysis. *Biol Neonate* 2005;87:27–34.
7. Wiswell TE, Gannon CM, Jacob J, Goldsmith L, Szyld E, Weiss K, et al. Delivery room management of the apparently vigorous meconium-stained neonate: results of the multicenter, international collaborative trial. *Pediatrics* 2000;105:1–7.
8. Vohra S, Roberts RS, Zhang B, Janes M, Schmidt B. Heat Loss Prevention (HeLP) in the delivery room: a randomized controlled trial of polyethylene occlusive skin wrapping in very preterm infants. *J Pediatr* 2004;145:750–3.
9. Edwards AD, Brocklehurst P, Gunn AJ, Halliday H, Juszczak E, Levene M, et al. Neurological outcomes at 18 months of age after moderate hypothermia for perinatal hypoxic ischaemic encephalopathy: synthesis and meta-analysis of trial data. *BMJ* 2010;340:c363.

26 Perinatal loss: management of late fetal death and stillbirth

Stillbirth is a common adverse pregnancy outcome, affecting 1/200 pregnancies. It often exerts profound emotional and psychological effects on parents, their relatives and friends. In the UK, stillbirth is defined as a baby delivered with no signs of life that is known to have completed at least 24 weeks of gestation. This definition is based on the fact that babies that reach this gestational age are usually viable. In the USA, where the gestational age threshold for stillbirth is lower (20 weeks if the gestational age is known, or weight at least 350 g if the gestational age is unknown), the incidence is 1/160 pregnancies, although this definition is not adopted by all states of the USA. The 350 g cut-off is the 50th centile for fetal weight at 20 weeks of gestation. The Australian definition specifies that fetal death is termed a stillbirth after 20 weeks of gestation or if the baby weighs more than 400 g. The World Health Organization defines stillbirths as fetal deaths in babies weighing 500 g or more or at a gestational age of 22 weeks or more. This definition applies to stillbirth figures from 1995 onwards. The term fetal death applies to babies with no signs of life in utero.

The overall stillbirth rate in the UK is 5.2/1000 total births, while the adjusted rate is 3.9/1000, with a regional variation ranging from 3.1 to 4.6/1000. These rates have remained largely static in the first decade of the 21st century despite improvements in perinatal care, prompting suggestions that rising average maternal age and obesity rates may be underlying causes of the lack of improvement. On the other hand, the stillbirth rate in the USA fell from 7.5/1000 births in 1990 to 6.2/1000 births in 2004.[1]

This chapter covers the causes of stillbirth, the immediate care and subsequent evaluation of the mother and the management of her future pregnancies, drawing on the authors' experience of running a dedicated perinatal loss service over a 10-year period. The reader is referred to more detailed reviews on perinatal loss counselling and psychological support, including the role of advocates, spiritual or religious leaders such as priests and imams, and support groups.

Risk factors for stillbirth

The most common risk factors associated with stillbirth in developed countries include black race, obesity, extremes of maternal age, comorbidities, smoking and substance misuse. Compared with their white counterparts, the stillbirth rates in 2007 for women of black and Asian ethnicity in the UK were 2.7 and 2.0 times higher, respectively.[2] This is also true for non-Hispanic black women in the USA, among whom the stillbirth rate is 11.25/1000 births compared with rates of ≤6/1000 births in Hispanic, non-Hispanic white, Asian and Native American women.[1] Ethnicity is associated with other risk factors, including deprivation, and should not be regarded as an independent variable.

Obesity remains an independent risk factor for stillbirth even after controlling for gestational diabetes, pre-eclampsia and smoking.[3] It is likely that other factors associated with maternal obesity, including social deprivation and specific comorbidities, contribute to stillbirths in this subset of women. Even so, obesity is associated with a five-fold increase in stillbirths linked to placental dysfunction. Pre-existing medical conditions such as diabetes, hypertension, collagen, renal and thyroid disorders are associated with increased risks of stillbirth. Family or personal history of thromboembolism or thrombophilias is also associated with an increased risk of stillbirth. While preconception optimisation of glucose may modify the risk of stillbirth,[4] there is no evidence that screening for thrombophilia modifies the risk of stillbirth or is cost-effective. Furthermore, pregnancy complications such as cholestasis, pre-eclampsia, multifetal gestations and infections with syphilis, *Listeria* or parvovirus B19 also increase the risk of stillbirth.

Aetiology of stillbirth

CHROMOSOMAL AND GENETIC ABNORMALITIES

Chromosomal abnormalities may be found in up to 13% of stillbirths, rising further to ≥20% in fetuses with anatomical malformations. These figures contrast with an incidence of 4.6% in normally formed fetuses.[5] Since karyotypic analyses of cell culture may fail in up to 50% of attempts, especially in fetuses with severe tissue autolysis, karyotypic analysis underestimates the role of genetic abnormalities in stillbirth. Furthermore, the contribution of single gene defects and micro-deletions to stillbirths is yet to be properly elucidated. Parents often receive the finding of a lethal chromosomal abnormality in a stillbirth with mixed feelings. Although it provides an explanation for their loss, it also raises anxiety about the risks of recurrence.

FETAL GROWTH RESTRICTION

There is a strong correlation between fetal growth restriction and the risk of stillbirth. The most severely affected fetuses (weight under the 2.5th centile) are at greatest risk. For example, the risk of fetal demise is approximately 1.5% at fetal weights below the 10th centile compared with 2.5% at weights below the 5th centile for gestational age.[6] Fetal growth restriction is notoriously difficult to define and characterise but is widely accepted to account for the majority of stillbirths.

PLACENTAL ABRUPTION

Placental abruption is a direct cause of fetal death and the pathway through which other contributors, including maternal substance abuse, smoking, pre-eclampsia and hypertension, exert their deleterious effects. Fetal demise is more likely if abruption occurs in the preterm fetus.

INFECTION

Infection is an important and well-documented cause of stillbirth in the preterm fetus, but its contribution to fetal loss at term is understated in the literature. In the authors' experience, subclinical chorioamnionitis and fetal sepsis are not infrequent causes of stillbirth. The pathogens responsible are usually enteropathogenic organisms including group B streptococcus (GBS), coliforms and anaerobes. In recent years the authors have observed an increase in the number of cases driven by other streptococcal strains such as *Streptococcus milleri*, *Staphylococcus* species and other sub-pathogenic organisms. The majority of cases are secondary to ascending infection, although we occasionally see vertical transmission of GBS from maternal sepsis. In our experience, fetal demise owing to *Listeria monocytogenes* or syphilis is exceedingly rare.

CORD EVENTS

Cord accidents may lead to fetal demise, but this diagnosis requires evidence of obstruction to blood flow such as is seen in true knots in the cord or circulatory compromise owing to umbilical or chorionic vascular thrombosis. The role of nuchal cord in the absence of the above features is dubious and other causes should be excluded first, before fetal death can be attributed to cord events.

Management

INITIAL MANAGEMENT

Effective management of the woman with a fetal death or stillbirth includes the provision of sensitive and supportive care for her and her family in an appropriate setting, preferably remote from other expectant or labouring mothers. Maternity units should ideally have a self-contained and secluded room(s) to manage labour and delivery in women with fetal death or those with intrapartum stillbirths.

If the woman was unaccompanied at the time of diagnosis, an offer should be made to contact her partner, relatives or even friends as appropriate. The woman's wishes around the timing of delivery should be explored. Although some women may wish to proceed promptly to delivery within minutes of the diagnosis of fetal death or even request a caesarean section, there is usually scope to allow one or two intervening days for them to come to terms with the loss. Much is made of the risk of coagulopathy with a retained dead fetus, but this risk is less than 10% within 4 weeks of diagnosis, rising to 30% thereafter in fetuses of 20 weeks of gestation or more. The woman's mode of delivery should be planned taking into consideration her obstetric history.

After the delivery of the baby, it is critically important to discuss and suggest tests aimed at determining the cause(s) of the fetal death, including a postmortem examination of the baby. During these discussions, clinicians should refer to the baby by name if one was given. Parents may decline autopsy on their baby for sentimental or religious reasons. This should be respected. It is not always possible for postmortem examination to determine the cause of fetal demise; however, parents should be sensitively informed that without an autopsy not only will the ability of the clinicians to find an explanation for their loss be limited, but they may also miss a key opportunity to offer the parents interventions that could prevent a recurrence in a future pregnancy. In our practice, we often see parents who revise their decision to decline a postmortem. Unfortunately, some of these grief-stricken parents were simply asked by the attending clinicians whether they wanted a postmortem examination or not without any explanation of the reasons for recommending one. A brief description of the postmortem procedure should be given, including a leaflet, and parents should be informed that their baby's face will not be disfigured during autopsy. Indeed, many pathologists access the baby's internal organs from the back and the cranial cavity posteriorly to disguise the signs of autopsy. If parents decline a full postmortem examination, a limited examination should be offered. This includes external examination, skin biopsy, blood tests, X-ray imaging, magnetic resonance imaging and photographs. In general, a limited postmortem is associated with less definitive results, and the role of magnetic resonance imaging as an alternative to postmortem examination is still under evaluation.

The woman's general practitioner and all her relevant healthcare providers should be informed of her loss to allow them to update their records and to prevent inappropriate queries about defaulting clinic appointments.

METHODS AND TIMING OF DELIVERY

For the overwhelming majority of women, vaginal delivery is the preferred mode of delivery, but caesarean section may be considered in a very small number of cases. Up to 90% of women will achieve vaginal delivery within 24 hours of induction of labour for fetal demise.[7] Vaginal delivery has the potential advantages of immediate recovery and shorter hospital stay. However, caesarean section may be indicated by virtue of maternal condition, or the woman herself may request a caesarean section because of previous experiences or a wish to avoid vaginal birth of a dead baby. This requires careful and sensitive discussion, with the implications of caesarean delivery for future childbearing discussed in detail.[8] In our practice, caesarean delivery for fetal demise is considered only in the most exceptional circumstances.

The RCOG recommends a combination of mifepristone and a prostaglandin preparation as first-line treatment for induction of labour in women with an unscarred uterus.[9] Mifepristone reduced the induction-to-delivery interval by approximately 7 hours when used in combination with misoprostol compared with regimens that did not include mifepristone.[7] Misoprostol (prostaglandin E_1) is preferred to prostaglandin E_2, although both preparations are equivalent in safety and efficacy. Misoprostol is cheaper and effective at lower doses, which are not currently available in the UK. Vaginal misoprostol is as effective as the oral form and is associated with fewer adverse effects such as diarrhoea, vomiting, shivering and pyrexia. The National Institute for Health and Clinical Excellence (NICE) has recently endorsed an RCOG recommendation that the dose of misoprostol should be adjusted according to gestational age: 100 micrograms 6-hourly before 26 weeks of gestation and 25–50 micrograms 4-hourly at 27 weeks of gestation or more.[10,11] The use of misoprostol in pregnancy is off-label in the UK and the lower doses are not available. Our own attempts to obtain lower doses of misoprostol from our local pharmacy has not been completely successful because the Medicines and Healthcare products Regulatory Authority advises against pharmacy departments removing tablets from blister strips to supply as stock, as this practice could interfere with the stability of the tablets. The current recommendation of the Society of Obstetricians and Gynaecologists of Canada is that misoprostol is contraindicated in women with previous caesarean delivery because of a high rate of uterine rupture; this is in contrast to the guidance issued by the RCOG and NICE in the UK in October 2010,[9–11] demonstrating that practice in this area is widely variable.

WOMEN WITH PREVIOUS UTERINE SCAR

The safety and benefits of induction of labour in women with previous caesarean scar and fetal death should be discussed in detail with the woman, preferably by a consultant obstetrician or a senior registrar acting in that capacity. Induction of labour with prostaglandin is safe in this context, but is not risk free. Misoprostol has been shown to be safe for induction of labour in women with a single previous lower-segment caesarean scar and a fetal death, but only at doses that are not currently available or marketed in the UK. Women with two previous caesarean scars may be reassured that the risk of induction of labour with prostaglandin is only marginally higher than that for women with a single previous scar. There are no reliable safety data on women with more than two caesarean scars or atypical scars. Mifepristone may be used alone to induce labour, thereby avoiding the use of prostaglandin, but the use of mifepristone in this context is also off-label. A randomised controlled trial of oral mifepristone alone (200 mg three times a day for 2 days) was compared with placebo in women with a fetal death. Labour occurred within 72 hours in significantly more women in the mifepristone group (63% compared with 17%, $P < 0.001$).[12]

Mechanical methods for induction of labour, such as a transcervical balloon catheter in women with a previous scar, have a special appeal as clinicians try to avoid the use of prostaglandin for induction of labour in women with uterine scars. The use of a transcervical balloon catheter after 28 weeks of gestation was associated with similar uterine rupture rates to spontaneous labour (0.55%) and significantly lower rates than prostaglandins (1.59%).[13] However, mechanical methods of induction might increase the risk of ascending infection in the presence of a fetal death and are not currently recommended in the UK for women with uterine scar and fetal demise outside the context of clinical trials.

ANALGESIA

All the usual modalities of analgesia during labour, including regional anaesthesia and patient-controlled anaesthesia, should be available to women with fetal death. Diamorphine and morphine have greater analgesic qualities and longer duration of action than pethidine and should be used in preference to pethidine. If the woman chooses to have regional anaesthesia, disseminated intravascular coagulation (DIC) and sepsis should be excluded before administering the anaesthetic.

MATERNAL EVALUATION

The mother should be thoroughly examined and investigated during the acute episode to assess maternal wellbeing and exclude potentially life-threatening maternal disease such as pre-eclampsia, chorioamnionitis or placental abruption. These conditions should be managed promptly if present. Details of events during the pregnancy and the results of investigations may indicate the possible cause of fetal death and the risk of recurrence, and may also assist clinicians in avoiding that risk. Women who choose expectant management should be informed of the risk of DIC, which is approximately 10% within 4 weeks of late fetal death ($\geq$20 weeks of gestation), rising to 30% thereafter. The onset of DIC should be monitored with twice-weekly clotting studies, platelet count and fibrinogen measurement until delivery occurs.

The aim of additional tests is to identify the cause of late fetal death and therefore answer the parents' question 'why?'. The tests should be comprehensive even if one cause is particularly suspected. In one study, about 95% of 314 women stated that it was important emotionally to have an explanation for their baby's death.[14] However, in almost 50% of stillbirths no specific cause is found, although there is an inverse relationship between gestational age at stillbirth and the chance of finding a cause. When a cause is found, it can crucially influence care in a future pregnancy. An abnormal result may be incidental and not necessarily linked to the fetal death; for example, factor V Leiden is present in about 5% of the general population and will often be an incidental finding.[15] Further tests might be indicated following the results of postmortem examination; for example, we would undertake parental thrombophilia screening and extended maternal glucose screening in a subsequent pregnancy if the postmortem examination revealed extensive thrombosis of fetal umbilical and/or chorionic vessels, villous immaturity and/or cherubic facies. We increasingly see postmortem reports showing classic pathological features of diabetes in stillborn infants where there had been no clinical evidence of disturbance of maternal glucose metabolism. Further research is required to understand this in greater detail.

COMMON CAUSES OF LATE FETAL DEATH

Antepartum and intrapartum causes:
- Placental abruption
- Maternal and fetal infection
- Cord prolapse
- Idiopathic hypoxia–acidosis
- Uterine rupture

Transplacental infections:
- Cytomegalovirus
- Syphilis
- Parvovirus B19
- *Listeria monocytogenes*
- Rubella
- Toxoplasmosis
- Herpes simplex
- Coxsackievirus
- Leptospira
- Q fever
- Lyme disease
- *Malaria parasitaemia*

Ascending infection, with or without membrane rupture:
- *Escherichia coli*
- Klebsiella
- GBS
- Enterococcus
- Mycoplasma/ureaplasma
- *Haemophilus influenzae*
- Chlamydia

Major fetomaternal haemorrhage may lead to fetal death from anaemia and hypovolaemia. A Kleihauer test should be performed in all women to exclude this cause of fetal death. In women who are rhesus D (RhD)-negative, the potentially sensitising bleed might have occurred days before the recognition of fetal death and time is of the essence to initiate anti-RhD immune globulin administration within the optimal window of 72 hours.[16] Although the benefit of anti-RhD is reduced when given beyond 72 hours, some benefit is still conferred up to 10 days after the sensitising event. A persistently positive Kleihauer test may be because the baby's blood group is also RhD-negative or because there has been a very large RhD-positive fetomaternal haemorrhage: it is important to distinguish between these two scenarios. If there has been a large fetomaternal haemorrhage, the dose of anti-RhD immune globulin should be adjusted upwards and the Kleihauer test should be repeated at 48 hours to ensure the fetal red cells have cleared.

An extended panel of thrombophilia tests (see box below) is recommended, especially in cases with severe placental pathology, severe growth restriction and in women with a personal or family history of thrombosis. The results may have implications for the management of any future pregnancy. Protein C and S activity is reduced by pregnancy and we would normally defer these tests for 3 months after delivery.

EXTENDED THROMBOPHILIA TESTS

- Anticardiolipin antibodies
- Lupus anticoagulant
- Factor V Leiden
- Prothrombin gene defects
- Methyl tetrahydrofolate reductase
- Antithrombin III levels
- Protein C activity
- Protein S activity

THE ROLE OF ASCENDING PERINATAL INFECTIONS

Ascending infection is a common cause of late fetal death and most probably contributes to a significant proportion of intrapartum fetal distress and neonatal encephalopathy in liveborn infants. Contrary to common belief, there is no requirement for prior rupture of fetal membranes. The usual organisms responsible include GBS, coliforms, anaerobes and organisms associated with bacterial vaginosis and aerobic vaginitis. In a significant minority of cases, no organisms are isolated despite histological evidence of severe chorioamnionitis and fetal host response to infection. This may be attributable to antenatal or intrapartum administration of antibiotics, culture techniques or the fact that the organisms are fastidious. The use of DNA amplification tests may be helpful in these cases. When placental swabs are taken, they should be obtained from the intramembranous space instead of the fetal or maternal surface. We recommend full genitourinary screening in these women and consider intermittent eradication of GBS in recurrent cases where this organism has been isolated from the fetal systemic circulation and shown to be the culprit. There is very slim evidence for this practice, but the principle is identical to decolonising GBS-positive women during labour to prevent fetal exposure. Occasionally, we encounter fetal death owing to common commensal organisms in association with membrane sweeping/stripping. We exercise due caution in these cases and do not recommend this procedure in subsequent pregnancies, especially when abnormal genital tract flora has been documented.

There is no role for routine antibiotic prophylaxis in women with fetal death or prophylaxis for those colonised with group B streptococcus, but women with signs of sepsis should be treated vigorously with intravenous broad-spectrum antibiotics including antichlamydial agents. The dead fetus can act as a focus for severe secondary infection including gas-forming clostridial species, which can result in severe sepsis and DIC.[17,18] It has been suggested that artificial rupture of membranes may facilitate ascending infection, although there are no prospective studies on this. It is likely that this link was made years ago when artificial rupture of membranes was the only method of induction of labour. Historically, and prior to the development of pharmacological agents for induction of labour, labour and delivery after fetal demise must have been prolonged and prone to infectious complications – and more so if the membranes were ruptured.

MANAGEMENT OF SUBSEQUENT PREGNANCY AFTER STILLBIRTH

Psychological support and reassurance are major parts of the care in a subsequent pregnancy after stillbirth. In our service, the women have direct telephone access to a specialist bereavement midwife and we are privileged to be able to offer them reassurance ultrasound scans on demand and growth scans every 4–5 weeks. During the preconception visit, weight loss and smoking cessation may be suggested. The test results and autopsy findings should be reviewed and a plan of care outlined in the notes. The woman's subsequent care should be provided by a limited number of carers. It is very disconcerting for women with a history of stillbirth to have to go over their history with a new or different doctor or midwife at every clinic attendance, and even worse when women are left with the impression that the clinician that attended to them did not know the details of their history or care.

Many of these women feel anxious around the time of their previous loss and may need extra support around this time. We do not routinely induce labour at 38 or 39 weeks of gestation if the baby is growing and developing normally and there are no maternal complications. Furthermore, we do not have a policy of routine induction of labour or delivery in the week before gestation of the previous loss. Instead, we individualise each case, discuss the situation with the woman, allay her fears and offer extra support and/or fetal surveillance, especially if the Bishop score is unfavourable. Sometimes, the woman may continue to be anxious and we have to proceed with the delivery.

Statutory requirements, administrative issues and documentation

The Births and Deaths Registration Act 1953, amended by the Still-Birth (Definition) Act 1992, sets out the legal definition of stillbirth as 'any child expelled or issued forth from its mother after the 24th week of pregnancy that did not breathe or show any other signs of life'. The guidance for practice is outlined below. Obstetricians and midwives should be aware of the law and statutory requirements related to stillbirth.

• A fully registered doctor or midwife who was present at the birth or examined the baby after birth must medically certify stillbirth. (Statute)

• HM Coroner must be contacted if there is doubt about the status of a birth. (Statute)

• Police should be contacted if there is suspicion of deliberate action to cause stillbirth. (Statute)

• The parents are responsible in law for registering the birth but can delegate the task to a healthcare professional. (Statute)

• Fetal deaths delivered later than 24 weeks that had clearly occurred before the end of the 24th week do not have to be certified or registered. (Code of Practice)

• The baby can be registered as indeterminate sex awaiting further tests. (Code of Practice)

The doctor or midwife attending the stillbirth is required to issue a Medical Certificate of Stillbirth that enables the birth to be registered. The certificate should include as much detail of the medical events leading to the fetal death as possible, but should avoid nonspecific medical terms such as anoxia and prematurity. The results of a post-mortem examination are not essential for certification. The parents, if married at the time of birth, are responsible for registering the stillbirth, normally within 42 days, but this responsibility can be delegated to healthcare professionals present at the birth or a bereavement support officer. If the couple were not married at the time of the birth, the responsibility for registering the stillbirth rests with the mother; the father's details may be added to the registration if he attends the registrar's office and signs the stillbirth register with the mother or makes a statutory declaration acknowledging his paternity (produced by the mother) or, where the mother is unable to go to the registrar's office with the father, the mother makes a statutory declaration acknowledging the father's paternity, which the father must produce to the registrar.

SPIRITUAL GUIDANCE, BURIAL AND CREMATION ISSUES

The legal responsibility for the child's body rests with the parents, but this can be delegated to hospital services. The parents should choose freely whether to hold or attend a funeral service. Having a funeral service for the infant was associated with slower resolution of women's psychological distress in one study.[19] Maternity units should have arrangements with elders of all common faiths and nonreligious spiritual organisations as a source of guidance and support for parents, and should provide a book of remembrance for parents, relatives and friends. If the parents request cremation, they have to complete the necessary cremation form, which is specific for a stillborn child, and follow the procedure.

Conclusions

Fetal death and stillbirth are common and are associated with marked physical and psychological morbidity. Appropriate management should aim to promptly identify and treat any complicating maternal morbidity, investigate the cause of the stillbirth and plan for any future pregnancy with a view to preventing recurrence. Furthermore, the service should offer avenues for spiritual and religious support as well as deal with the legal and statutory requirements around stillbirth.

References

1. MacDorman MF, Munson ML, Kirmeyer S. Fetal and perinatal mortality, United States, 2004. *Natl Vital Stat Rep* 2007;56:1–19.
2. Confidential Enquiry into Maternal and Child Health. *Perinatal Mortality 2007*. London: CEMACH; 2009 [http://www.cmace.org.uk/Publications-Press-Releases/Report-Publications/Perinatal-Mortality.aspx].
3. Cnattingius S, Stephansson O. The epidemiology of stillbirth. *Semin Perinatol* 2002;26:25–30.
4. Karlsson K, Kjellmer I. The outcome of diabetic pregnancies in relation to the mother's blood sugar level. *Am J Obstet Gynecol* 1972;112:213–20.
5. Korteweg FJ, Bouman K, Erwich JJ, Timmer A, Veeger NJ, Ravisé JM, et al. Cytogenetic analysis after evaluation of 750 fetal deaths: proposal for diagnostic workup. *Obstet Gynecol* 2008;111:865–74.
6. Getahun D, Ananth CV, Kinzler WL. Risk factors for antepartum and intrapartum stillbirth: a population-based study. *Am J Obstet Gynecol* 2007;196:499–507.
7. Wagaarachchi PT, Ashok PW, Narvekar NN, Smith NC, Templeton A. Medical management of late intrauterine death using a combination of mifepristone and misoprostol. *BJOG* 2002;109:443–7.

8. National Collaborating Centre for Women's and Children's Health, National Institute for Health and Clinical Excellence. *Caesarean section.* Clinical Guideline. London: RCOG Press; 2004 [http://www.nice.org.uk/CG013].

9. Royal College of Obstetricians and Gynaecologists. *Late Intrauterine Fetal Death and Stillbirth.* Green-top Guideline No. 55. London: RCOG; 2010 [http://www.rcog.org.uk/womens-health/clinical-guidance/late-intrauterine-fetal-death-and-stillbirth-green-top-55].

10. Gómez Ponce de León R, Wing D, Fiala C. Misoprostol for intrauterine fetal death. *Int J Gynaecol Obstet* 2007;99 Suppl 2:S190–3.

11. National Collaborating Centre for Women's and Children's Health, National Institute for Health and Clinical Excellence. *Induction of labour.* Clinical Guideline. London: NICE; 2008 [http://www.nice.org.uk/guidance/CG70].

12. Cabrol D, Dubois C, Cronje H, Gonnet JM, Guillot M, Maria B, et al. Induction of labor with mifepristone (RU 486) in intrauterine fetal death. *Am J Obstet Gynecol* 1990;163:540–2.

13. Al-Zirqi I, Stray-Pedersen B, Forsén L, Vangen S. Uterine rupture after previous caesarean section. *BJOG* 2010;117:809–20. Erratum: *BJOG* 2010;117:1041.

14. Rådestad I, Nordin C, Steineck G, Sjögren B. A comparison of women's memories of care during pregnancy, labour and delivery after stillbirth or live birth. *Midwifery* 1998;14:111–7.

15. Rees DC, Cox M, Clegg JB. World distribution of factor V Leiden. *Lancet* 1995;346:1133–4.

16. Fox R. Preventing RhD haemolytic disease of the newborn. RhD negative women who have intrauterine death may need anti-D immunoglobulin. *BMJ* 1998;316:1164–5.

17. Catanzarite V, Schibanoff JM, Chinn R, Mendoza A, Weiss R. Overwhelming maternal sepsis due to a gas-forming *Escherichia coli* chorioamnionitis. *Am J Perinatol* 1994;11:205–7.

18. Braun U, Bearth G, Dieth V, Corboz L. [A case of disseminated intravascular coagulation (DIC) in a cow with endometritis and fetal death]. *Schweiz Arch Tierheilkd* 1990;132:239–45. Article in German.

19. Hughes P, Turton P, Hopper E, McGauley GA, Fonagy P. Factors associated with the unresolved classification of the Adult Attachment Interview in women who have suffered stillbirth. *Dev Psychopathol* 2004;16:215–30.

Index

audit 4, 41
augmentation of labour 16–17, 20, 148, 173, 178, 258
autopsies 276–7

B-Lynch sutures 219–20
bacterial vaginosis 86
Bakri balloons 215–16
balloon catheters
  for cervical ripening 77, 278
  for uterine tamponade 215–16
bearing-down effort 20–1
beta-agonists 90, 91, 247
betamethasone 92–3, 94
bilateral shoulder dystocia 117–18, 125, 127–8
bladder
  caesarean sections 158, 165
  cord compression 191, 193
  hysterectomy 183
  placenta percreta 203, 204
  uterine rupture 173–4
bleeding see haemorrhage
blood pressure see hypertension; hypotension
blood transfusions 207–8, 240, 242
brachial plexus injuries 119, 121
bradycardia
  fetal 35, 173
  neonatal 256
Braxton Hicks bipolar podalic version 202
breathing
  apnoeic neonates 262
  neonatal resuscitation 263–7, 269, 270
breech delivery
  caesarean 133, 161, 245, 248
  in multiple pregnancy 148–50, 153
  vaginal 133–42
breech extraction in caesarean sections 166
broad-ligament haematomas 71

caesarean sections 155–66
  anaesthesia 156, 193

antibiotics 156
breech fetuses 133, 161, 245, 248
classical 157–8, 163–5, 169–70, 203
in cord compression 192–4
with deeply engaged fetal head 165–6
documentation 166
in fetal death 277
increase in numbers of 155
indications for 155–6, 199, 208
low vertical 157, 159, 165, 170
lower transverse segment 157, 158–63, 170, 173, 200
in multiple pregnancy 145, 152, 153, 161
in placenta praevia 199, 200–1
in placenta praevia accreta 203, 204
in pre-eclampsia 258
repeat 170, 171
in shoulder dystocia 121, 127–8, 156
thromboprophylaxis 157
after trial of assisted vaginal delivery 104–5, 112–13
vaginal delivery after 80–1, 169–74, 278
calcium channel blockers 91, 256
calcium gluconate 255
caput 22, 103
carbetocin 57
carboprost (15-methyl prostaglandin F2α) 57, 213
cardiac compression, neonatal 268
cardiopulmonary resuscitation
  maternal 235
  neonatal 261–71
cardiotocography (CTG) 25, 30, 32–3
  admission 14, 34
  induction of labour 79
  interpretation 34–41, 48, 94, 173
central venous pressure 257
cephalic replacement 127–8, 246, 248

rhesus prophylaxis 198, 280–1
risk factors
    PPH 211–12
    preterm labour 85–6
    shoulder dystocia 120–1
    stillbirth 274
    uterine rupture 80–1, 169–71,
        177–8, 182
risk management 4–5
ritodrine 90
rotational forceps 108–10

SBAR tool (patient handover) 6
scalp electrodes 32
seaweed 76
shock
    in PPH 214
    in uterine inversion 226, 227
shoulder dystocia 117–29, 156, 170,
    246
sodium bicarbonate 269
square compression sutures 220–1
ST waveform analysis 44–7
stabilising induction 81
staff 2–3, 282
steroids
    in amniotic fluid embolism 235
    for improving fetal lung
        maturity 90, 92–3, 94
    progesterone in preterm labour
        86–7
stillbirth 273–84
    definition 273, 283
    disposal of the body 284
    epidemiology 273
    freshly stillborn babies 262, 272
    legal requirements 283
    management 74, 81–2, 276–82
    risk factors and causes 274–5,
        280
    subsequent pregnancies 282
    see also perinatal mortality rates
stimulation tests 47
supralevator haematomas 71
suturing techniques
    anal sphincter trauma 68–9
    arterial ligation 216–17

caesarean sections 162–3, 165,
    170–1
    episiotomy 64–5
    uterine compression 219–21
    vaginal lacerations 67
symphysiotomy 128
Syntometrine 56–7

tachycardia
    fetal 35, 40, 173, 247
    maternal 247, 256
tamponade, uterine 200, 215–16
terbutaline 247
Term Breech Trial 133
term prelabour rupture of
    membranes (term PROM) 95–6
thrombocytopenia 242, 254, 257,
    259
thrombophilia 281
thromboplastin release 207, 240
thromboprophylaxis 157
tocography 32, 33
    see also cardiotocography (CTG)
tocolytic drugs/tocolysis
    acute 245–8
    breech delivery by caesarean
        section 161, 245
    prevention of preterm birth
        90–2
    retained placenta 59, 60, 246
    twin deliveries 147, 246
    uterine inversion 227, 246, 248
training and education 4
transcervical balloon catheters 77,
    278
transvaginal ultrasound 87, 197
transverse lie 148–50, 161
triplets 145, 152–3
turtle sign 122
twins see multiple pregnancy

ultrasound
    cervical length and preterm
        labour 87
    fetal heart rate 32
    placenta praevia 197, 198
    vasa praevia 205